THE BODYBUILDING
COOKBOOK

100 DELICIOUS RECIPES TO BUILD MUSCLE, BURN FAT AND SAVE TIME

JASON FARLEY

Copyright

Legal Disclaimer

The information in the book is for educational purposes only. It is not medical advice and is not intended to replace the advice or attention of health-care professionals. Consult your physician before beginning or making any changes in your diet or exercise program. Specific medical advice should be obtained from a licensed health-care practitioner. Jason Farley and his associates will not assume any liability, nor be held responsible for any injury, illness or personal loss due to the utilization of any information contained herein.

CONTENTS

It's the most important meal of the day. Your parents told you. Your teachers told you. And now you know it. How can you expect not to have a total burn out, or beat your PB, or even have the energy to get your ass off the sofa if you haven't fuelled the machine? You can't. So use these quick, easy and tasty recipes to get you going.
And no, it's not all raw eggs…

Chicken breast and eggs. The first things you might be mistaken to think you have to subject yourself to for breakfast, lunch and dinner for the rest of your muscle-building life. But there is so much more out there within the chicken and poultry meal options. We all know chicken is great – it's low in fat and high in protein and we all know it's tasty so read on and find out how chicken and other poultry members can be exciting and effective in your meal-plan diary.

RED MEAT AND PORK 43

I've teamed pork with red meat because it has every bit as much macho power! Pork doesn't have to be dry and fatty it can be delicious with the recipes to follow. Red meat speaks for itself in the muscle building world – a slab of steak comes to anybody's mind when they are trying to get big! Hopefully from the next section I can provide you with alternative dishes to fill you up with iron, protein and much more!

A lot of us reserve fish for the refined. Either that or we're scared of cooking it. Fish is often easier than cooking meat; it's fresh, healthy and full of omega 3. Hopefully the recipes provided in this section will either get you started with cooking up fish, or further you down the chef road you're already on. oh, and it will mean you burn fat, build strength, and increase brain power all at the same time!

SALADS 76

Salads are boring right? They're only designed for rabbits and skinny women on diets. Wrong. Salads done right are firstly delicious and don't have to just be a side; secondly they can be stuffed with fibre, protein, vitamins, and nutrients. Don't make the stupid error of ignoring our age-old, trusted training companions and try a super strong salad soon.

Not enough to fill you up? Craving your side order of fries? Eyes bigger than your belly? No sweat. Here's a sweet collection of side orders you can prepare in your own home – add calories, protein and a little extra something, whilst knowing you've made it in the healthy way.

HOMEMADE PROTEIN SHAKES 98

If you want to spend hundreds of pounds on pre-made shakes full of chemicals and fillers that cements onto your kitchen sink then be my guest! If not, try these homemade healthy alternatives that will pack on just as much punch as the shop-bought varieties.

DESSERTS 117

Who's saying you can't indulge in a sneaky treat? I'm saying you can, and you can do it without the guilt with the recipes I've provided. Your sweet tooth need not be suppressed with these mouth-watering dishes. Go ahead – treat yourself! You need the calories after all…

CONVERSION CHARTS 129

Use a different method of measuring? No worries - I've got you covered!

BONUS CONTENT: THE BODYBUILDING COOKBOOK MEAL PLANS 133

I believe that anyone can build a fantastic body and to ensure you get there, I created The Fast and Fresh Bodybuilding Cookbook Meal Plans as a counterpart to this cookbook to save you the hard work when it comes to what to eat, how much to eat and when to eat. This special manual contains 6 different delicious daily meal plans ranging from 1500 calories all the way to a whopping 4000 calories, so you're in control of how big or shredded you wanna get!

WOULD YOU MIND DOING ME A FAVOR? 134

OTHER BOOKS BY ME... 135

With my books, I want to educate and support you in your quest to achieve all of your fitness goals. Whether you want to build muscle or burn fat and get shredded, there's something here for you. All of my books provide proven, sound training and nutritional advice backed by science (no bro-science here!)
And you won't need a fancy gym membership, tons of money or expensive supplements to be successful with my books - just the desire and willpower to change your life!

WELCOME

First off, I'd like to thank you for purchasing my book - *The Bodybuilding Cookbook.*

Within the following pages lies your complete nutritional toolkit for creating tasty muscle building meals that can be used to build muscle and burn fat!

Eating the right kind of foods is vital for anyone who wants to build muscle or get lean but it doesn't mean it has to be boring. So many athletes subject themselves to dull, bland meals, which becomes tedious, dull and repetitive over time. I created this book to teach you that it doesn't have to be that way. In this cookbook, you will find just over 100 delicious, mouth-watering ways to build muscle and burn fat.

This book will show you how you can whip up recipes that are not only healthy, but are also easy to prepare; thus, saving you a lot of precious time. In today's busy world, the ability to prepare quick and healthy meals will give you a decided advantage.

Each recipe also includes the exact amount of calories and the amount of protein, carbohydrates and fats you will get from each serving. The more higher calorie meals will be better suited to someone looking to build muscle and the lower calorie meals will be better suited to someone looking to burn fat. You won't need much equipment to make these recipes, at most a blender and a few pots and pans.

If you have been turned off by a lot of healthy bodybuilding meals that you have tried before, and are convinced that it is the price you have to pay to achieve your desired body, you are mistaken. The recipes you will find in this book are guaranteed to satisfy even the most discriminating taste buds.

Without further ado, grab your apron and let's get cooking!

Enjoy your meals,

Jason

MUSCLE IS WON OR LOST IN THE KITCHEN

Many experts feel that your nutritional habits make for up to 80% of the way your body looks. Every drip of sweat and effort you exude in the gym is wasted if your nutrition is not on point. If you want to build a substantial amount of muscle and strength or lose fat then you must fuel your body accordingly.

EATING FOR MUSCLE

To build muscle, you need to take in an excess of calories with the right nutrients to grow. If you don't eat enough, your body won't be able to fully repair the damage you cause by lifting weights, triggering you to plateau or even worse, lose muscle. However don't make the mistake most gym rats make by eating everything in sight, from pizzas to pop-tarts, as this is extremely unhealthy in the long-term. As you'll see from the upcoming recipes, eating the right foods doesn't have to be boring, bland or time–consuming.

EATING TO SHRED

To lose fat, you need to take in fewer calories than you expend. Again if you don't take in the right nutrients and foods, you will lose muscle. Losing fat generally requires you to be more precise which leads to many adopting the "Chicken, Rice and Broccoli diet," which is incredibly boring, bland and usually leads to many people failing.

I created these recipes to escape the tedious, boring diets that many gym-goers subject them-selves too and finally make dieting enjoyable.

THE FUNDAMENTAL PILLARS OF A MUSCLE BUILDING / FAT BURNING DIET

Before you ask, you won't need to be a qualified nutritionist to create your perfect diet. You just need to understand a few simple things:.

1. What Protein, Carbohydrates and Fats are and what they're used for.
2. How much to get of each and what foods to get them from.
3. How many calories you need to achieve your goals (Build Muscle or Burn Fat.)

WHAT IS PROTEIN?

Protein is used by your body for a number of processes from enzyme and hormone production to ensuring your immune system is working optimally. The reason why protein is so important in a muscle building diet is because protein is absolutely critical for muscle growth and repair. Working out and 'tearing down muscle' increases your body's demand for protein. As you build more and more muscle, the more protein your body will require to repair, grow and maintain that muscle. If you don't supply your body with enough protein, it will take it from your muscles causing muscle breakdown. Making sure you get enough protein is therefore of upmost importance in planning your diet.

WHAT ARE CARBOHYDRATES?

Carbohydrates get converted into glucose and then are used by your body for energy. There are two types of carbohydrates - simple and complex. Simple carbohydrates are foods like fruit, white rice and sugar. Complex carbohydrates are foods like sweet potatoes, brown rice and vegetables. Complex carbohydrates tend to be thought of as the better of the two. The difference between these types of carbohydrates is how long it takes the body to convert them into glucose. Simple carbohydrates are converted by your body quickly making them great for a fast source of energy however there is usually a fast decline after. It takes your body a lot longer to convert complex carbohydrates into glucose making them a much more sustaining source of energy. The reason so many people are afraid of carbohydrates is because whatever your body doesn't use gets moved into your fat stores. Carbohydrates however are not the enemy and are vital for your success.

WHAT ARE FATS?

Fats are vital for many of your bodily functions. They are needed for the production of many hormones in your body and they also help keep your brain and nervous system running optimally. They are also the most calorically dense out of the three macronutrients – every gram of fat contains 9 calories!
There are four types of fat: Monounsaturated, Polyunsaturated, Saturated and Trans-fatty acids. The only one you need to avoid is Trans-Fatty acids. These are fats that have been modified in a lab to ensure a longer shelf life. The body does not know what to do with them and therefore they can get into your cells and cause damage. They're most commonly found in packaged meals and used in many fried foods.

How much do you need of each? Well that depends on your goals!

TO BUILD MUSCLE, A GOOD PLACE TO START FROM IS:

Protein = 1.5 grams per pound of bodyweight
Carbohydrates = 2 grams per pound of bodyweight
Fats = 0.5 grams per pound of bodyweight

You want to be gaining about 0.5 – 1 pound a week. Any more than that and you will be gaining too much fat. If you find you aren't gaining weight, increase your calories by around 100-200 calories each week until you reach the sweet spot. Alternatively if you're gaining too much, then you want to reduce your calories by around 100 – 200 each week.

TO MAINTAIN MUSCLE, A GOOD PLACE TO START FROM IS:

Protein= 1 gram per pound of bodyweight
Carbohydrates = 1 gram per pound of bodyweight
Fats = 0.5 grams per pound of bodyweight

TO LOSE WEIGHT, A GOOD PLACE TO START FROM IS:

Protein = 2 grams per pound of bodyweigh,
Carbohydrates = 0.5 grams per pound of body-weight
Fats = 1 gram per pound of bodyweight

You want to be losing about 1 – 2 pound a week. Any more than that and you risk losing that hard earned muscle. If you find you aren't losing weight, decrease your calories by around 100-200 calories each week until you reach the sweet spot. Alternatively if you're losing too much, then you want to increase your calories by around 100 – 200 each week.

THE TOP COMMANDMENTS OF GOOD NUTRITION

What you put into your body will either make or break the results you get in the gym. These are rules you must live by if you want to be successful in your muscle building and fat loss pursuits.

1. HAVE PROTEIN WITH EVERY MEAL

Protein is vital to your success if building or maintaining muscle mass is your goal. Aim to have a least 1 source of quality protein with every meal. At a minimum, you must aim for at least 1 pound of protein per pound of bodyweight.

2. THERE MUST BE GREEN ON THE PLATE

Vegetables contain so many essential nutrients that you simply can't get anywhere else. Aim to have at least 1 serving of vegetables with every meal.

3. FAT IS NOT EVIL

Lets get one thing straight; fat will not make you fat. If you want to build muscle and burn fat, it's vital that you get enough. As we've established, healthy fats are needed for the production of many hormones in your body including testosterone. The only fats you need to avoid are trans fats.

4. DON'T RELY ON SUPPLEMENTS, EAT (REAL) FOOD

Supplements are meant to supplement your diet not make up the bulk of it. Aim to have at least 70% of your diet come from "real" food.

5. STICK TO SLOW DIGESTING CARBS MOST OF THE TIME (EXCEPT AROUND YOUR WORKOUTS)

Slow digesting carbohydrates ensure a steady supply of energy and have less of an impact on your blood sugar levels. Regular consumption of fast digesting carbs has been linked to an increased risk of diabetes, heart disease and obesity. However after training, you want to replace your depleted glycogen stores quickly as this can prevent your body becoming catabolic and keep you in a "muscle building" state. This is why you would want to consume a fast digesting carbohydrate after your workout.

6. DRINK WATER AND LOTS OF IT

It is absolutely essential to drink enough water. When you don't get enough, performance can be severely affected. Therefore try to get in about 3 – 4 litres of pure, clean water per day.

BREAKFAST

It's the most important meal of the day. Your parents told you. Your teachers told you. And now you know it. How can you expect not to have a total burn out, or beat your PB, or even have the energy to get your ass off the sofa if you haven't fuelled the machine? You can't. So use these quick, easy and tasty recipes to get you going. And no, it's not all raw eggs…

MASS BUILDING
SWEET POTATO PANCAKES

Start your day with this quick and easy, delicious protein packed pancake recipe. It contains all the right ingredients to keep you going and more than enough protein for your muscles to feast on!

CALORIES PER SERVING: 451

PROTEIN: 38G

CARBS: 74G

FAT: 9G

SERVES 1

1 medium sized sweet potato

1 egg

4 egg whites

100g of fat-free Greek yogurt

40g of oats

1 tsp cinnamon

1 tsp vanilla extract

Handful of diced strawberries

Handful of blueberries

1 tsp of honey

HOW TO MAKE:

Rinse sweet potato under cold water for a couple of seconds and then pierce it with a fork several times and place it in the microwave until soft (about 8 minutes).

After let it cool down before removing all skin with a knife.

Put the oats into a blender and blend until they are a fine powder, then place into a bowl.

Place the sweet potato in the blender and blend until smooth, and then mix with the powdered oats.

Add the egg, egg whites, vanilla, cinnamon, honey and yogurt and stir well. This is now your pancake batter.

Spray a pan with cooking spray and place over medium heat. Pour roughly a quarter of the batter into the pan and cook for 1-2 minutes.

Flip the pancake and cook for another 30 seconds. Once done, remove your tasty pancake and top with the berries. Use the same method for the rest of your batter.

BRAWNY
BREAKFAST BURRITO

Add a bit spice to your life with this Mexican inspired burrito. Contains great sources of protein, healthy fats and fibre to ensure you're building muscle the lean way.

CALORIES PER SERVING: 302

PROTEIN: 25G

CARBS: 19G

FAT: 16G

SERVES 1

2 eggs

50ml of low fat milk

25g of black beans

50g of low fat cheese

Handful of chopped red peppers

1tsp of chopped coriander

1tbsp of salsa

½ a tsp of cumin

HOW TO MAKE:

Add the milk, eggs and cumin to a bowl and whisk together.

Spray pan with cooking spray and place over medium heat. Add the mixture to the pan.

After roughly 2 – 3 minutes, add the low fat cheese, chopped red peppers and black beans to the omelette.

Once added fold the omelette in half and let it cook through (1-2 minutes).

Remove from pan and serve with the salsa and coriander.

SUPER SCRAMBLED TURKEY BACON EGGS ON TOAST

Mix up your boring egg based breakfasts with this delicious recipe. Eggs are a great source of complete protein as they contain all eight amino acids.

CALORIES PER SERVING: 299

PROTEIN: 22G

CARBS: 35G

FAT: 8G

SERVES 2

6 egg whites

3 slices of turkey bacon

2 slices of Ezekiel bread

Handful of chopped onion

Handful of chopped peppers

Handful of chopped white mushrooms

1tsp of garlic powder

1tsp of dried parsley

1tsp of olive oil

HOW TO MAKE:

Spray pan with cooking spray and place over medium/high heat. Add the chopped onions, chopped yellow peppers and white mushrooms and cook until soft.

In a different pan, cook the turkey bacon.

Add the egg whites and garlic powder to the pan with the veggies and 1tsp of olive oil and scramble until the eggs become firm.

Toast the Ezekiel bread.

Break up the turkey bacon and add to the scrambled eggs

Plate up and serve scrambled eggs and turkey bacon on bread, sprinkled with the fresh parsley.

Add salt and pepper as required.

BANANA AND ALMOND MUSCLE OATMEAL

If you're in a hurry, this recipe is great. It takes around 5 minutes to make and still has the right macro-nutrients to make this a healthy and sustaining meal.

CALORIES PER SERVING: 523

PROTEIN: 32G

CARBS: 60G

FAT: 15G

HOW TO MAKE:

Throw the oats and low fat milk into a large bowl and place in the micro-wave for two minutes.

Add the diced banana, peanut butter, whey protein and chopped almonds to the oats and mix in.

SERVES 1

50 grams of rolled oats

200ml of low fat milk

1 scoop of whey protein (vanilla or chocolate)

Handful of chopped almonds

1tsp of organic peanut butter

1 diced banana

PROTEIN POWERED PANCAKES

If you're not a fan of sweet potato, then these are a great alternative. Lots of protein and quick and easy to make.

CALORIES PER SERVING: 337

PROTEIN: 27G

CARBS: 33G

FAT: 9G

MAKES 5 PANCAKES

6 egg whites

40g of rolled oats

1 tsp flaxseed oil

1 tsp of cinnamon

1 tsp of stevia

HOW TO MAKE:

Put the oats and all the other ingredients into a blender and blend. This is now your pancake batter.

Spray pan with cooking spray and place over medium heat.

Pour roughly 1/5 of the pancake batter into the pan and cook for 1-2 minutes. Flip the pancake and cook for another 30 seconds.

Once done, remove your tasty pancake.

Use the same method for the rest of your batter.

TURKEY
MUSCLE OMELETTE

If you're looking for a protein packed, low carb meal for breakfast then this is it. Contains 26 grams of protein and only 5 grams of carbs.

CALORIES PER SERVING: 358

PROTEIN: 26G

CARBS: 5G

FAT: 21G

SERVES 2

150g of chopped or minced turkey

3 eggs

Handful of baby spinach

Handful of kale

1 tbsp of olive oil

25g of low fat cheese

HOW TO MAKE:

Crack the eggs into a bowl and whisk.

Grab a pan and heat half the oil on a medium heat, then add the turkey, kale and cheese and cook for 5-6 minutes.

In a different pan, heat the rest of the olive oil and then add the eggs and cook for around 4 minutes.

Add the turkey mix into the pan with the eggs and sprinkle some baby spinach on top, then fold the omelette in half.

Cook for another 2-3 minutes.

Plate up and serve.

AESTHETIC
ASPARAGUS FRITTATA

A high protein, low carb breakfast. Great for those looking to minimize their carb intake

CALORIES PER SERVING: 349

PROTEIN: 23G

CARBS: 8G

FAT: 25G

SERVES 3

300g of chopped asparagus

½ broccoli (florets only)

8 eggs

Handful of chopped parsley

1 tsp of chives

1 tbsp of olive oil

100ml of low fat milk

Salt and pepper

HOW TO MAKE:

Crack the eggs into a bowl, add the milk and some salt and pepper and whisk.

Get a covered skillet and steam the broccoli over a medium heat for 4-5 minutes. Set to one side.

Next, in the same skillet, heat the oil. Add the chopped asparagus, chopped parsley and chives into the skillet and cook for around 2-3 minutes on a medium heat.

Add the egg mixture, along with the broccoli into the skillet and cover the skillet evenly.

Cook for around 3-4 minutes or until the eggs are set right through

Take the skillet and place under the grill for around 2 minutes or until the top is golden (optional).

Plate up and serve.

POWER
PROTEIN WAFFLES

Who said waffles are unhealthy? My waffle recipes are packed full of protein and without the guilt on the side!

CALORIES PER SERVING: 314

PROTEIN: 37G

CARBS: 28G

FAT: 5G

HOW TO MAKE:

Add all the ingredients into a blender and blend.

Add the mixture to a waffle iron and bake.

SERVES 2

4 eggs whites

1 scoop of vanilla protein powder

40g of rolled oats

1 tsp of baking powder

½ tsp of stevia

SCRAMBLED EGGS WITH SPINACH

Tasty, quick and easy breakfast packed full of protein!

CALORIES PER SERVING: 282

PROTEIN: 23G

CARBS: 15G

FAT: 15G

SERVES 2

3 eggs

5 egg whites

1 cup of baby spinach

50g of grated low fat cheese

Handful of chopped onion

Handful of chopped red peppers

1 tsp of olive oil

HOW TO MAKE:

Spray pan with cooking spray and place over medium/high heat.

Add the chopped onions, chopped red peppers and cook until soft.

Add the egg and egg whites to the pan with the veggies with 1tsp of olive oil and scramble until the eggs become firm.

Sprinkle the baby spinach leaves and cheese over the eggs.

Plate up and serve scrambled eggs.

Add salt and pepper as required.

CHICKEN AND POULTRY

Chicken breast and eggs. The first things you might be mistaken to think you have to subject yourself to for breakfast, lunch and dinner for the rest of your muscle-building life. But there is so much more out there within the chicken and poultry meal options. We all know chicken is great – it's low in fat and high in protein and we all know it's tasty so read on and find out how chicken and other poultry members can be exciting and effective in your meal-plan diary.

SWEET
HONEY AND CHILLI CHICKEN DRUMSTICKS

Add a little sweet and savoury kick to your favourite protein source.

CALORIES PER SERVING: 479

PROTEIN: 42G

CARBS: 17G

FAT: 27G

SERVES 1

6 chicken drumsticks

Sprinkle of salt and pepper

2 tbsp of sesame oil

1 diced red pepper

1 finely diced chilli

1 tbsp of organic honey

3 minced garlic cloves

HOW TO MAKE:

In a bowl, add the honey, chilli, garlic, diced red pepper, sesame oil, salt and pepper.

Mix them together.

Pour half of the honey mixture over the chicken drumsticks.

Make sure that the drumsticks are covered evenly.

Leave the chicken mix to marinate for at least 3 hours or overnight if possible.

Preheat the grill to a medium heat when ready.

Line a baking tray with tin foil and spread the chicken out evenly.

Grill under a medium heat for 25-30 minutes.

Check chicken is cooked through and piping hot before serving.

Plate up and serve.

(Tastes great with my "Muscle Rice Salad" pg 93)

ANABOLIC
JERK CHICKEN AND BROWN RICE

Add a little spice to your life with this traditional Caribbean dish. Packed full of protein and slow releasing carbohydrates to keep to you growing.

CALORIES PER SERVING: 516

PROTEIN: 32G

CARBS: 76G

FAT: 33G

SERVES 1

100g of chicken thighs or breast	½ of dried thyme
½ tsp of ground allspice	1 chopped onion
½ tsp of black pepper	2 scotch bonnet chillies
½ tsp of nutmeg	1/2 chopped red pepper
½ tsp of cinnamon	60g of brown rice
½ tsp of sage	1 tsp of olive oil
½ tsp of dried thyme	
1 clove of garlic	

HOW TO MAKE:

To make the jerk paste, add the allspice, nutmeg, sage, cinnamon, dried thyme, garlic, red pepper, black pepper, onion, olive oil and scotch bonnet chillies to the blender and blend until it's a puree.

Rub the paste over the chicken breasts and leave them for at least one hour to marinade.

Add the chicken breasts to the grill and grill them for roughly 10-12 minutes per side or until they are cooked through. Put to one side once cooked.

Meanwhile add 300ml of cold water to a pot and heat until the water is boiling. Once boiling, add the rice and leave for 20 minutes.

Drain the rice and serve with the chicken.

LAZY CHICKEN
AND EGG STIR FRY

This meal is quick to prepare and contains two great protein sources to build muscle and burn fat.

CALORIES PER SERVING: 409

PROTEIN: 46G

CARBS: 89G

FAT: 20G

SERVES 1

100g of chopped chicken breast

2 eggs

100g of brown rice

2 tsp of chinese five spice

100g of Mixed frozen veg

HOW TO MAKE:

Add 300ml of cold water to a pot and heat until the water is boiling. Once boiling, add the rice and leave for 20 minutes. Drain the rice and place to one side.

Heat a pan on a medium heat and add the chopped chicken and spices.

Stir-fry for roughly 5 minutes.

While the chicken is cooking, boil or steam the frozen veg for 5 minutes until cooked and beat the eggs in a separate bowl.

Add the rice and beaten eggs to the pan with the chicken and stir until the eggs start to scramble 3-4 minutes.

Finally add the veg to the pan and stir for a further 2-3 minutes

Plate up and serve.

POWER
PESTO CHICKEN PASTA

Great protein packed pasta dish to mix things up!

CALORIES PER SERVING: 550

PROTEIN: 25G

CARBS: 30G

FAT: 19G

SERVES 2

200g of chopped grilled chicken breast

100g of whole-wheat pasta

1 tbsp of pesto

A pinch of black pepper

Handful of basil

Handful of spinach

Handful of rocket

Handful of pine nuts

Handful of diced tomatoes

2 tbsp of olive oil

HOW TO MAKE:

Heat a large pan of water on high until it boils.

Add the whole-wheat pasta and leave until the water returns to boiling point.

Reduce the heat until the water simmers. Leave the whole-wheat pasta to cook for around 10 minutes.

Get a bowl and add the pesto, olive oil and black pepper and mix together.

Add the chopped chicken breast, pine nuts, tomatoes and herbs to the mixture.

Drain the pasta and fold the mix into the pan until the pasta is covered.

MUSCLE
MOROCCAN CHICKEN CASSEROLE

This meal is quick to prepare and contains two great protein sources to build muscle and burn fat.

CALORIES PER SERVING: 409

PROTEIN: 46G

CARBS: 89G

FAT: 20G

SERVES 1

4 chicken breasts

1 tsp of ground cumin

1 tsp of paprika

1 tbsp of olive oil

1 chopped onion

350g of canned chopped tomatoes

2 tbsp harissa paste

1 tbsp honey

2 medium thickly sliced courgettes

400g of drained and rinsed chickpeas

A pinch of salt and pepper

HOW TO MAKE:

Sprinkle salt, pepper, paprika and the ground cumin over the chicken breasts.

Then grab a large pan and add the olive oil and heat on a medium heat.

Add the chicken and onions to the pan and cook the chicken for roughly four minutes per side.

Pour the chopped tomatoes into the pan along with 200ml of water and add the honey, harissa, courgettes and chickpeas and stir the ingredients together.

Bring the mix to a simmer and then leave to cook for around 15 minutes.

Plate up and serve.

BRAWNY CHICKEN & CHORIZO JAMBALAYA

A very tasty muscle-building recipe, inspired from Cajun cuisine. Contains a good helping of protein and slow releasing carbs to keep you burning fat and building muscle.

CALORIES PER SERVING: 286

PROTEIN: 30G

CARBS: 61G

FAT: 14G

SERVES 4

2 chopped chicken breasts

1 chopped onion

1 chopped red pepper

2 crushed garlic cloves

100g chorizo, sliced

1 tbsp Cajun seasoning

250g brown rice

1 tbsp olive oil

350g of tinned chopped tomatoes

350ml chicken stock

HOW TO MAKE:

Grab a large pan and add the olive oil and heat on a medium heat.

Add the chicken and brown for around 8 minutes. Place to one side.

Add the onion to the pan and fry until tender. Get the garlic, chorizo, Cajun seasoning and red pepper and add to the pan and cook for around 5 minutes.

Add the brown rice along with the chopped tomatoes, chicken and chicken stock to the pan. Cover the pan and let simmer for around 25 minutes or until the rice is soft.

SPICY
CHICKEN TRAY-BAKE

A very simple to make chicken recipe that tastes great and contains all the necessary muscle building nutrients.

CALORIES PER SERVING: 276

PROTEIN: 40G

CARBS: 14G

FAT: 7G

SERVES 4

4 skinless chicken breasts

3 tbsp harissa paste

250g of low-fat natural yogurt

1 small, chopped and peeled butter-nut squash

2 chopped red onions

1 tbsp olive oil

HOW TO MAKE:

Pre-heat oven (375°F/190 °C/Gas Mark 5).

Add 3 tbsp of yogurt and 2 tbsp of the harissa to a bowl and mix together. Coat the chicken breast with the mixture and leave to one side.

Add the onions, chopped butternut squash, 1 tbsp of harissa and 2 tbsp of olive oil to a tray and place in the oven and cook for around 10 minutes.

Take the tray out of the oven and add the chicken breast to the tray. Place back in the oven and cook for around 20 minutes until the chicken is cooked right through.

Plate up and serve with the leftover yogurt.

HEALTHY
TURKEY BURGERS

Get your burger fix with this healthy turkey alternative.

CALORIES PER SERVING: 362

PROTEIN: 38G

CARBS: 39G

FAT: 7G

SERVES 4

500g of mince turkey

1 onion, finely chopped

1 chopped romaine lettuce

4 wholemeal buns

2 diced tomatoes

1 crushed garlic clove

1 lemon

3 tbsp grated parmesan

Chopped parsley

3 tbsp low-fat Greek yogurt

HOW TO MAKE:

Pre-heat oven (375°F/190 °C/Gas Mark 5).

In a bowl, add the crushed garlic, 2 tbsp of parmesan and parsley.

Cut the lemon in half and squeeze the lemon juice over the ingredients.

Mix all the ingredients together.

Add the ingredients to the minced turkey along with the onion and mix them together.

Using your hands, mould the mince mixture into 4 burgers and place on a tray and then cook for around 20 minutes or until the burgers have cooked right through.

While the burgers are cooking, cut open the whole-wheat buns and mix the yogurt with the lettuce. Add the burgers to the buns along with the yogurt-lettuce mixture and tomatoes.

TURKEY MEATBALL FIESTA

Healthy turkey meatballs with added oats to keep you building muscle and burning fat.

CALORIES PER SERVING: 315

PROTEIN: 35G

CARBS: 23G

FAT: 10G

SERVES 4

500g of turkey mince	1 tsp olive oil	3 tsp chipotle chilli paste
50g porridge oats	1 chopped red onion	300ml chicken stock
2 chopped spring onions	2 chopped garlic cloves	400g of canned chopped tomatoes
1 tsp ground cumin	1 large chopped yellow pepper	400g of drained black beans
1 tsp coriander	1 tsp ground cumin	1 avocado, stoned, peeled and chopped
Handful of chopped coriander		

HOW TO MAKE:

Add the mince to a bowl with the oats, chopped spring onions, spices and coriander and mix together.

Mould the mince mixture into 12 small 'meatballs' using your hands.

Add some olive oil to the pan on a medium heat; add the meatballs and cook them until golden.

Take them from the pan and leave to one side.

Add the onion, chopped pepper and chopped garlic to the pan and cook until tender.

Add the chilli paste and ground cumin and chicken stock to the pan and stir well. Then add the meatballs back into the pan.

Cover and cook on a low/medium heat for around 10 minutes.

Add the tomatoes and black beans to the pan and cook uncovered for around 2-3 minutes.

Serve with the chopped avocado and coriander.

ANABOLIC RATATOUILLE CHICKEN

A tasty low-carb chicken recipe to keep you building muscle and burning fat.

CALORIES PER SERVING: 324

PROTEIN: 38G

CARBS: 10G

FAT: 15G

SERVES 4

4 chicken breasts

1 chopped onion,

2 chopped red peppers

1 courgette, cut into chunks

1 small aubergine, cut into chunks

4 chopped tomatoes

4 tbsp of olive oil

A pinch of salt and pepper

HOW TO MAKE:

Pre-heat oven (375°F/190 °C/Gas Mark 5).

Add all the vegetables and the tomatoes to a tray and drizzle with 3 tbsp. olive oil.

Place the chicken breasts over the vegetables and season with the remaining tbsp of olive oil and some salt and pepper.

Place the tray in the oven and cook for around 30 minutes.

Plate up and serve

BRAWNY CHICKEN CHASSEUR

A classic, tasty chicken dish that's packed with protein and low carbs.

CALORIES PER SERVING: 242

PROTEIN: 50G

CARBS: 5G

FAT: 3G

SERVES 4

8 chopped rashers of turkey bacon

4 chopped chicken breasts

200g of baby mushrooms

1 tbsp plain flour

400g of canned chopped tomatoes

1 beef stock cube

Worcestershire sauce

Handful of chopped parsley

Olive oil

HOW TO MAKE:

Heat the olive oil on a medium heat in a shallow saucepan and add the turkey bacon and cook for 4-5 minutes until it starts to brown.

Add the chopped chicken breasts and cook for around 5 minutes until golden. Increase the heat to high and add the baby mushrooms for 2 minutes. Add the flour and stir in until a paste starts to form.

Add the canned chopped tomatoes and beef stock cube to the saucepan and cook for around 10 minutes.

Then add the parsley and Worcestershire sauce to the pan, stir in and then serve.

AESTHETIC
TOMATO AND OLIVE PAN-FRIED CHICKEN

A tasty chicken dish that's sure to satisfy your hunger and nutritional needs.

CALORIES PER SERVING: 334

PROTEIN: 39G

CARBS: 8G

FAT: 19G

SERVES 2

2 Chicken breasts

1 chopped onion,

2 chopped garlic cloves

400g of canned chopped tomatoes

1 tbsp balsamic vinegar

6 chopped green olives

300ml chicken stock

2 tbsp olive oil

Handful of basil leaves

A pinch of salt and pepper

HOW TO MAKE:

Heat olive oil on a medium heat in a pan.

Sprinkle some salt and pepper over the chicken and then place the chicken in the pan and cook for roughly 10 minutes, or until the chicken has cooked right through..

Add the onion to the pan and turn the chicken over and cook for another 4 – 5 minutes. Remove the chicken from the pan and place to one side.

Add the garlic to the pan and continue to cook the onions until tender.

Add the chopped tomatoes, olives, chicken stock and balsamic vinegar to the pan with most of the basil leaves and turn down the heat, simmering for around 8 minutes.

Place the chicken back into the pan, cover and simmer for a further 5 minutes

Plate up and serve with the remaining basil as a garnish.

CHICKEN BRAWN BURGER

Another great healthy burger alternative! Quick and easy to make if you're strapped for time. Contains a good helping of protein to keep you anabolic.

CALORIES PER SERVING: 458

PROTEIN: 50G

CARBS: 38G

FAT: 12G

SERVES 1

1 chicken breast

1 tbsp low fat mayonnaise

1 chopped red onion

1 chopped lettuce

1 slice of low-fat cheddar

1 whole wheat burger bun

1 tsp of chopped jalapeno

Olive oil

HOW TO MAKE:

Heat olive oil on a medium heat in a griddle pan.

Cover the chicken breast with some salt and pepper and add to the pan and cook for around 5 minutes. Turn it over and cook for a further 5 minutes.

Add the slice of cheddar to the top of the chicken. Cook chicken for another 8 minutes or until chicken is cooked right through.

Remove chicken from pan and place to one side.

Cut open the roll and add the chicken, onions, mayonnaise, lettuce and chopped jalapeno

.

GRILLED
CHICKEN AND RED ONION SKEWERS

A power-protein snack, contains a whopping 73 grams of protein!

CALORIES PER SERVING: 488

PROTEIN: 73G

CARBS: 10G

FAT: 17G

SERVES 1

2 chicken breasts

2 minced garlic cloves

1 chopped red chilli (deseeded)

2 tbsp of sesame oil

1 red onion, chopped into eight pieces

Sprinkle of salt and pepper

3 wooden skewers

HOW TO MAKE:

Chop the chicken breasts into chunky pieces using a sharp knife or scissors.

Mix the sesame oil with the minced garlic, chilli and salt and pepper (as desired).

Marinate the chicken in half the oil and leave for at least one hour - if possible leave to marinate overnight.

Keep the rest of the oil for brushing whilst cooking.

Heat the grill to a high heat and soak wooden skewers in water.

Take skewers from the water and pierce a chunk of chicken followed by a slice of red onion – repeat this until skewer is covered.

Grill for 15-20 minutes, using a brush to rub the remaining oil over the chicken every five minutes and turning throughout.

Check there is no pink inside the chicken when cut and that it is boiling hot before serving).

DICED
CHICKEN WITH EGG NOODLES

Mix things up with this tasty recipe. Contains the right amount of protein, carbs and fats to meet your goals.

CALORIES PER SERVING: 322

PROTEIN: 30G

CARBS: 31G

FAT: 8G

SERVES 2

150g of chopped chicken breast

50g of egg noodles

1 grated carrot

2 tbsp of fresh orange juice

1 tsp of sesame seeds

3 tsp of soy sauce

1 tsp of rapeseed oil

1 chopped ginger

100g of sugar snap peas

HOW TO MAKE:

Heat 1 tsp rapeseed oil on a medium heat in pan.

Cook the chopped chicken breast for about 10-15 minutes or until cooked through.

While cooking the chicken, place the noodles in a pot of boiling water for about 5 minutes.

In a bowl, mix together the ginger, sesame seeds, soy sauce, 1 tsp rapeseed oil and orange juice.

Once chicken is cooked and noodles are cooked and drained, add the chicken, noodles, carrot and peas to the dressing and mix

HONEY
GLAZED GROWTH CHICKEN

Mix things up with this sweet and tempting chicken recipe

CALORIES PER SERVING: 195

PROTEIN: 37G

CARBS: 9G

FAT: 2G

SERVES 2

2 chicken breasts with skin

½ lemon

1 tbsp honey

1 tbsp dark soy sauce

A pinch of salt and pepper

HOW TO MAKE:

Pre-heat oven (375°F/190 °C/Gas Mark 5).

Place the chicken breast on a baking dish and add a sprinkle of salt and pepper.

Get a bowl and squeeze the lemon juice in and add the honey and soy sauce. Mix the ingredients together and cover the chicken breasts with it.

Place the squeezed lemon in between the chicken breasts and place the dish into the oven and cook for around 30 minutes on until fully cooked through.

MIGHTY
MEXICAN CHICKEN STEW

Spice things up with this classic Mexican chicken stew. Packed full of protein from the chicken as well as the quinoa!

CALORIES PER SERVING: 464

PROTEIN: 51G

CARBS: 53G

FAT: 4G

SERVES 4

4 skinless chicken breasts

140g quinoa

400g of drained pinto beans

1 tbsp olive oil

1 chopped onion

2 chopped red peppers

3 tbsp chipotle paste

800g of tinned chopped tomatoes

2 chicken stock cubes

Handful of chopped coriander

1 lime

HOW TO MAKE:

Heat olive oil on a medium heat in a deep pan and add the onion and peppers and cook for 2-3 minutes.

Then add the chipotle paste and the tinned chopped tomatoes.

Add the chicken breast and add just enough water to cover the chicken by 1cm and then bring down the heat to let the mixture simmer. Cook for around 20 minutes until the chicken is cooked right through.

Add boiling water to a separate saucepan along with stock cubes. Pour in the quinoa and heat for around 12 minutes.

Add the pinto beans and cook for a further 3 minutes. Drain the quinoa and add in the coriander and squeeze the lime juice in - mix and place to one side.

Serve the chicken with the quinoa and cover with the tomato sauce from the pan.

SPICY
CAJUN CHICKEN WITH GUACAMOLE

Tasty low fat, low carb chicken recipe. Contains a generous amount of protein to keep you building muscle and burning fat.

CALORIES PER SERVING: 190

PROTEIN: 34G

CARBS: 2G

FAT: 5G

SERVES 4

4 chicken breasts

1 tbsp paprika

1 tsp dried onion flakes

¼ tsp cayenne pepper

2 tsp dried thyme

Salt

Pepper

1 tbsp olive oil

200g of guacamole

HOW TO MAKE:

Get a bowl and add the cayenne pepper, dried thyme, paprika, salt, pepper and onion flakes and mix together.

Get the chicken and cut two deep scores on each breast. Rub the oil onto the chicken then cover the breasts with the spices.

Add the chicken to the grill and cook for around 8 minutes each side or until completely cooked through.

Serve chicken with the guacamole

MUSCLE
CHICKEN CACCIATORE

An Italian inspired, delicious, low fat, low carb chicken recipe. Contains a liberal amount of protein to keep you building muscle and burning fat.

CALORIES PER SERVING: 172

PROTEIN: 33G

CARBS: 6G

FAT: 2G

SERVES 4

4 chicken breasts

1 chopped onion

2 sliced garlic cloves

Salt

Pepper

1 tsp olive oil

400g of tinned chopped tomatoes

2 tbsp chopped rosemary leaves

Handful of basil leaves

HOW TO MAKE:

Pre-Heat oven (375°F/190 °C/Gas Mark 5).

Heat oil in a pan on a medium heat and add the onion and garlic and cook until soft.

Pour in the chopped tomatoes, rosemary, salt and pepper and cook for around 15 minutes until the mixture has become thicker.

Spread the mixture over the chicken; place the chicken on a tray and transfer to the oven. Leave in the oven for 20 minutes until the chicken is cooked right through. Sprinkle the basil over the chicken and serve

RED MEAT AND PORK

I've teamed pork with red meat because it has every bit as much macho power! Pork doesn't have to be dry and fatty it can be delicious with the recipes to follow. Red meat speaks for itself in the muscle building world – a slab of steak comes to anybody's mind when they are trying to get big! Hopefully from the next section I can provide you with alternative dishes to fill you up with iron, protein and much more!

SUPER
HERBY LAMB STEAKS

A succulent lamb dish, helping you to enjoy the taste of bulking.

CALORIES PER SERVING: 308

PROTEIN: 34G

CARBS: 15G

FAT: 14G

SERVES 2

2x 400g lamb leg steaks or
equivalent weight

2 chopped zucchinis (courgettes)

2 tbsp olive oil

50g arugula (rocket)

2 garlic cloves, chopped

8 halved baby cherry tomatoes,

Handful of chopped cilantro
(coriander)

Sprinkle of salt and pepper

HOW TO MAKE:

Preheat the grill to a medium to high heat.

Add the oil to a pan and heat on a heat.

Throw in the courgettes, tomatoes and garlic and fry until courgettes and
tomatoes are soft.

Stir in the arugula and cilantro.

Meanwhile, sprinkle some salt and pepper over the lamb steaks.

Place the lamb on a baking tray and grill for 4 minutes each side.

Plate and serve with the roasted vegetables.

ANABOLIC PORK SOUP

This soup is quick to prepare and full of protein to build muscle and burn fat.

CALORIES PER SERVING: 297

PROTEIN: 21G

CARBS: 13G

FAT: 17G

SERVES 4

400g diced pork steaks

600ml chicken stock

1 tbsp soy sauce

2 tsp Chinese five-spice powder

25 ginger finely chopped

200g pack of baby spinach

1 tsp of chopped red chilli,

200g of rice noodles

Handful of chopped spring onions

HOW TO MAKE:

Get a large saucepan and add all the ingredients except for the spring onions and noodles. Cover the pan and bring to a simmer on a medium heat.

Without letting the ingredients boil, leave to cook for around 8-10 minutes.

While cooking the pork, place the rice noodles in a pot of boiling water for about 5 minutes and then drain.

Drain and place the noodles in a bowl and add the pork and greens over the noodles. Sprinkle the spring onions over the dish and serve.

POWER
PORK FRUIT TRAY

This dish is absolutely delicious and one of my favourite pork recipes. Contains a good helping of protein and is low on carbs for those of you who are shredding!

CALORIES PER SERVING: 335

PROTEIN: 42G

CARBS: 12G

FAT: 14G

SERVES 4

4 pork steaks

1 tbsp olive oil

2 diced red onions

2 chopped large pears

Small handful of rosemary

50g diced blue cheese

1 diced couchette

Handful of pine nuts

HOW TO MAKE:

Get a large pan and heat the olive oil on a medium heat.

Add the courgette, red onions, chopped pears, salt and pepper.

Fry for around 6 minutes until the veg starts to caramelise.

Pre-heat the Grill.

Get a cooking tray and transfer the ingredients along with the rosemary sprigs to the tray. Sprinkle some salt and pepper over the pork steaks and place them in the tray.

Place the tray in the oven and grill for around 10-15 minutes or until cooked right through, turning the pork steaks half way through. Add the cheese and pine nuts and let the cheese melt for a further 4-5 minutes.

Plate up and serve.

MUSCLE BUILDING
STEAK & SWEET POTATO FRIES

A great, healthy alternative to regular steak and chips. Contains a good helping of protein and slow releasing carbs.

CALORIES PER SERVING: 418

PROTEIN: 29G

CARBS: 39G

FAT: 15G

SERVES 4

100g of sirloin steak

200g of sweet potatoes cut into chips

1 tbsp olive oil

1 chopped red onion

1 bag of pre-washed salad

1 tbsp of balsamic vinegar

A pinch of black pepper

HOW TO MAKE:

Pre-Heat oven (375°F/190 °C/Gas Mark 5).

Get a baking tray, spread the chips out and bake for around 25 minutes.

While the chips are cooking, get a large frying pan and heat the olive oil on a medium heat.

Pepper the steaks and add to the pan. Fry the steaks for 6 minutes in total, turning the steaks once halfway through.

Take the steak and leave to cool.

Get a large bowl and add the salad and chopped onion. Drizzle with the vinegar and serve with the potatoes and steak.

ORIENTAL
BEEF MUSCLE STIR-FRY

Great beef recipe, packed with loads of protein to keep you growing and burning fat.

CALORIES PER SERVING: 349

PROTEIN: 34G

CARBS: 26G

FAT: 14G

SERVES 4

500g of diced beef rump,

1 tsp Chinese five-spice powder

300g of egg noodles

1 large chopped red chilli

1 chopped garlic clove

1 chopped ginger

1 stick lemongrass

2 tbsp of olive oil

100g sugar snap peas

8 baby corn, sliced diagonally

6 chopped spring onions

½ lime

2 tbsp soy sauce

1 tbsp fish sauce

2 tbsp roasted peanuts

1 chopped coriander, to serve

HOW TO MAKE:

Get a bowl and add the beef and five-spice and leave to marinade. Place the egg noodles in a pot of boiling water for about 5 minutes, drain and then place to one side.

Mix together the chopped chilli, ginger, garlic and lemongrass in a bowl.

Add 1 tbsp of olive oil to a wok and heat on a medium heat. Add the ginger mixture into the wok and fry for 1 minute. Turn up the heat and add 1 more tbsp of olive oil to the wok and add the beef and fry until browned.

Add the sugar snaps, spring onions and baby corn to the wok and continue to stir-fry for around a minute before adding the egg noodles and mix together. Turn off the heat and add the soy sauce, fish sauces and squeezed lime juice.

Place in a bowl and add the peanuts and chopped coriander to serve.

BRAWNY
BEEF FAJITAS

Quick and easy beef recipe, perfect for lunch, packed with loads of protein to keep you growing and burning fat.

CALORIES PER SERVING: 358

PROTEIN: 28G

CARBS: 40G

FAT: 10G

HOW TO MAKE:

Add the diced steak, chopped onion, red pepper and 1 tbsp of chilli sauce to a pan and stir fry for around 4 – 5 minutes.

Place the wrap in the microwave for 30 seconds

Add the steak mix to the fajita and along with one more tbsp of sweet chilli sauce, roll up and enjoy

SERVES 1

100g of diced lean steak

1 chopped red onion

1 chopped red pepper

1 wholegrain fajita wrap

2 tbsp of sweet chilli sauce

BULK-UP
LAMB CURRY & PEANUT STEW

This absolutely delicious curry is packed full of flavour and has a hefty does of protein to boot.

CALORIES PER SERVING: 600

PROTEIN: 44G

CARBS: 38G

FAT: 46G

SERVES 4

50g chopped peanuts

400ml can coconut cream

4 tbsp massaman curry paste

600g diced lamb steak (or beef)

450g chopped white potatoes

1 chopped onion

1 cinnamon stick

1 tbsp tamarind paste

1 tbsp fish sauce

1 sliced red chilli

HOW TO MAKE:

Pre-heat oven (375°F/190 °C/Gas Mark 5).

Get a large casserole dish and place on the gas/electric hob on a medium heat.

Add 2 tbsp of coconut cream and the curry paste and fry for around a minute before adding the diced lamb. Stir in and brown. Add the rest of the coconut cream with a cup of water as well as the potatoes, onions, cinnamon stick, tamarind, fish sauce and peanuts.

Reduce heat to a simmer, cover the casserole, transfer to the oven and cook for 2 hours until the lamb is soft and tender.

Add the sliced chilli to the top and serve.

MIGHTY LAMB CASSEROLE

This absolutely delicious curry is packed full of flavour and has a hefty does of protein to boot.

CALORIES PER SERVING: 380

PROTEIN: 35G

CARBS: 33G

FAT: 9G

SERVES 2

1 tbsp of olive oil

2 cubed lamb fillets

1 chopped onion,

2 chopped carrots, thickly sliced

Handful of kale

400ml of chicken stock

1 tsp dried rosemary

1 tsp of chopped parsley

400g of rinsed and drained cannellini beans

HOW TO MAKE:

Get a large casserole dish and heat the olive oil on a medium heat.

Add the lamb to the casserole dish and cook for 5 minutes until browned, then add the chopped onion and carrots. Leave to cook for another 5 minutes until the vegetables begin to soften.

Add the chicken stock, kale and rosemary. Then cover the casserole, leave to simmer on a low heat for 1-1.5 hours until the lamb is tender and fully cooked through.

Add the cannellini beans 15 minutes before the end of the cooking time.

Plate up and serve with the chopped parsley to garnish.

STEAK & CHEESE MUSCLE CLUB

A very quick and easy, tasty, healthy homemade sandwich with a generous amount of protein to ensure you continue to build muscle and burn fat.

CALORIES PER SERVING: 336

PROTEIN: 32G

CARBS: 27G

FAT: 11G

SERVES 2

1 250g sirloin steak

2 whole-meal bread rolls

1 tsp olive oil

1 tsp Dijon mustard

Handful of rocket

30g Stilton cheese

1 tsp of balsamic vinegar

A pinch of salt and pepper

HOW TO MAKE:

Heat up a griddle pan on a high heat until very hot. Drizzle the olive oil over the steak over both sides of the steak. Sprinkle some salt and pepper over it and place the steak in the pan and fry for 3 minutes on each side.

Place the steak to one side and leave to rest for a minute.

Cut in half to form two slices of steak.

Cut the whole-wheat rolls in half and place toast. Once done, add the mustard and rocket to the roll and place 1 half of the steak on top. Add balsamic vinegar and the cheese to the top and then make the sandwich.

Repeat steps with the other roll.

MASS GAINING LAMB FLATBREAD

A tasty and healthy homemade flatbread with a Moroccan twist, including a generous amount of protein to fuel you and your muscles!

CALORIES PER SERVING: 391

PROTEIN: 29G

CARBS: 34G

FAT: 17G

SERVES 4

2 200g lamb leg steaks

1 tbsp harissa

4 whole meal flatbreads

4 tbsp of organic houmous

Handful of baby spinach

Handful of watercress

A pinch of salt and pepper

HOW TO MAKE:

Preheat the grill.

Sprinkle harissa, salt and pepper over the lamb.

Place lamb on a baking tray and grill for 4 minutes before turning the lamb over and cooking for a further 4 minutes. Take the tray out of the grill and leave to one side.

Place the flatbreads under the grill for around 1 – 2 minutes before removing and spreading on the houmous.

Cut the lamb into thin strips and place over the flat bread.

Add the baby spinach and watercress, roll the flatbread into a wrap and enjoy.

SUPER STEAK, SPICY RICE & BEANS

The perfect steak...

CALORIES PER SERVING: 650

PROTEIN: 48G

CARBS: 60G

FAT: 26G

SERVES 2

2 250g sirloin steaks

4 tsp olive oil

1 small onion, sliced

100g brown long-grain rice

1½tsp fajita seasoning

1 can of drained kidney beans

Handful of chopped coriander leaves

2 tbsp tomato salsa, to serve

HOW TO MAKE:

Pour 3 tsp of oil into a deep saucepan on a medium heat and add the onion. Fry the onion for around 4 minutes.

Then add ½ the fajita seasoning and long grain rice. Cook for 1 minute. Add 300ml of boiling water to the saucepan and stir in. Cover the saucepan and let simmer for 20 minutes until the water has been absorbed and the rice is fluffy. Add the kidney beans and keep the pan warm.

While the rice is cooking, sprinkle salt and pepper over the steak as well as ½ fajita seasoning. Pre-heat a griddle pan on a high heat, add the steaks and cook for 8 minutes in total, turning the steaks half way through.

Add the rice to a bowl and mix in the coriander. Add a tbsp of tomato salsa to each of the steaks and serve.

MUSCLE
MINT LAMB STEAKS

Delicious recipe with over 40g of protein to keep you building muscle and burning fat.

CALORIES PER SERVING: 367

PROTEIN: 41G

CARBS: 2G

FAT: 22G

HOW TO MAKE:

Get a bowl and add the mint, vinegar and garlic and mix together.

Add the lamb to the bowl and leave to marinade for at least 30 minutes.

Pre-heat a griddle pan on a medium to high heat and cook the lamb for 4 minutes each side or until cooked through.

Serve alone or with your choice of salad for a delicious accompaniment.

SERVES 2

4 200g lamb leg steaks

2 tbsp olive oil

2 chopped garlic cloves

1 tbsp balsamic vinegar

Handful of chopped mint leaves

SUPER
LAMB STEAKS WITH MEDITERRANEAN VEG

A mediterranean twist on a lamb dish! A very quick and easy, healthy lamb recipe to keep you going for longer...

CALORIES PER SERVING: 308

PROTEIN: 34G

CARBS: 15G

FAT: 14G

HOW TO MAKE:

Add the oil to a pan and heat. Throw in the courgettes, tomatoes and garlic and fry until courgettes and tomatoes are soft. Add the rocket and coriander and stir in.

Meanwhile, sprinkle some salt and pepper over the lamb steaks. Place the lamb on a tray and grill for 4 minutes each side. Serve with the veg.

SERVES 2

2 lamb leg steaks

2 chopped courgettes

2 tbsp olive oil

Handful of rocket

2 garlic cloves, chopped

8 halved baby cherry tomatoes,

Handful of chopped coriander

STRENGTH AND MASS MEATLOAF

The perfect muscle building meatloaf!

CALORIES PER SERVING: 410

PROTEIN: 47G

CARBS: 15G

FAT: 19G

SERVES 6

900g of lean ground beef

1 tsp olive oil

1 chopped red onion

1 tsp garlic

3 chopped tomatoes

1 whole beaten egg

100g of whole wheat bread crumbs

Handful of parsley

20g of low fat parmesan

50ml of organic skim milk

A pinch of salt and pepper

1 tsp oregano

HOW TO MAKE:

Preheat the oven to (400°F/200 °C/Gas Mark 6).

Add the oil to a pan and heat on a medium heat.

Cook the onions until soft but not browned. Remove the onions from the pan and let cool.

Get a big bowl and mix all of the ingredients together.

Put the meat in a big baking tray and cook on a high heat for around 30-35 minutes.

Serve once cooked through and piping hot.

FARLEY'S
MUSCLE BUILDING CHILLI CON CARNE

Who doesn't like Chilli con carne? Well this healthy version will provide you with over 30g of protein and a smug sense of satisfaction!

CALORIES PER SERVING: 389

PROTEIN: 37G

CARBS: 25G

FAT: 17G

SERVES 4

500g lean ground beef

1 tbsp oil

1 chopped onion

1 chopped red pepper

2 crushed garlic cloves,

1 tsp of chilli powder

1 tsp paprika

1 tsp ground cumin

1 beef stock cube

400g of tinned chopped tomatoes

2 tbsp tomato purée

400g of dried and rinsed red kidney beans

100g of brown rice

HOW TO MAKE:

Get a pan and add the olive oil and heat on a medium heat.

Add the onions to the pan and fry until soft.

Then add the garlic, red pepper, chilli powder, paprika and cumin. Stir together and cook for 5 minutes.

Add the ground mince to the pan and cook until browned.

Get 300ml of hot water and add the beef stock cube to it. Add this to the pan along with the chopped tomatoes. Also add the puree and stir in well. Bring the pan to a simmer, cover and cook for around 50 minutes. Stir occasionally.

After 30 minutes and while the mince is cooking, add 300ml of cold water to a separate pot and heat until the water is boiling. Once boiling, add the rice and leave for 20 minutes.

Once the rice is done, drain and put to one side. Add the beans to the meat mix and cook for another 10 minutes.

Serve the rice topped with the chilli con carne.

TASTY
BEEF BROCCOLI STIR-FRY

A very quick and easy, healthy beef stir-fry that will save you reaching out for the local Chinese delivery menu!

CALORIES PER SERVING: 277

PROTEIN: 30G

CARBS: 7G

FAT: 14G

SERVES 4

400g of diced frying beef steaks

1 head of broccoli, broken into florets

4 chopped celery sticks

Handful of sweet corn

150ml beef stock

2 tbsp of horseradish sauce

1 tbsp of olive oil

A pinch of salt and pepper

HOW TO MAKE:

Heat the olive oil on a medium/high heat in a frying pan.

Add some salt and pepper to the beefsteaks and place in the frying pan.

Stir-fry for 2 minutes until the beef is browned then remove and set aside.

Add the broccoli and chopped celery to the pan and fry for a further 2 minutes.

Add the beef stock to the pan, then cover. Reduce the heat and let the veg simmer for 2 minutes.

Place the steak back in the pan and mix with the other vegetables for another minute.

Plate up and serve with the horseradish sauce.

FISH AND SEAFOOD

A lot of us reserve fish for the refined. Either that or we're scared of cooking it. Fish is often easier than cooking meat; it's fresh, healthy and full of omega 3. Hopefully the recipes provided in this section will either get you started with cooking up fish, or further you down the chef road you're already on. Oh, and it will mean you burn fat, build strength, and increase brain power all at the same time!

MUSCLE
MACKEREL AND SPICY COUSCOUS

Mackerel is a great healthy source of protein and is also a great source of omega-3 fats.

CALORIES PER SERVING: 484

PROTEIN: 26G

CARBS: 35G

FAT: 26G

HOW TO MAKE:

Pour the couscous into a bowl and add the cumin, smoked paprika and pinch of black pepper. Then grab a cup of boiling water and pour it over the couscous until it covers it by about 1cm. Cover the bowl and leave for around 10-15 minutes.

When the water has been absorbed, add the chopped chilli, chopped tomatoes, chopped mint and chopped onion to the bowl and stir.

Add the mackerel to the top and serve.

SERVES 1

150g of couscous

100g of pre cooked mackerel

1tsp of ground cumin

1 tsp of smoked paprika

1 chopped red chilli

Pinch of black pepper

2 chopped tomatoes

1 chopped onion

Handful of chopped mint

SUPER COD AND VEG

A simple recipe that's quick and easy to make and tasty too. You guessed it - high in protein and low in carbs!

CALORIES PER SERVING: 324

PROTEIN: 28G

CARBS: 11G

FAT: 19G

SERVES 1

140g fillet of white fish (Boneless)

1 cup of frozen peas

Salt

Pepper

1 tbsp of olive oil

2 sliced spring onions

1 chopped gem of lettuce

1 tbsp reduced-fat crème fraîche

HOW TO MAKE:

Add the lettuce, spring onions, frozen peas and olive oil to a microwave-proof bowl.

Season the fish with salt and pepper and 1 tbsp crème fraîche and add to the bowl.

Cover the bowl with cling film; pierce it several times with a fork and place in microwave.

Microwave the bowl for around 8 minutes until the fish as been fully cooked and is piping hot throughout.

Take the bowl from the microwave and remove the fish, placing to one side.

Use a fork to mash the vegetables and serve topped with the fish and an extra spoonful of crème fraîche.

LEMONY SALMON

Salmon is a great source of protein and is very high in omega 3 fats. Most salmon dishes can be bland and boring...Not this one!

CALORIES PER SERVING: 205

PROTEIN: 20G

CARBS: 1G

FAT: 13G

SERVES 4

4 100g Salmon fillets

1 lemon

A pinch of salt and pepper

10g of chopped tarragon

Handful of rocket

2 tbsp of olive oil

1 chopped garlic clove

HOW TO MAKE:

Pre-Heat grill.

Get a bowl and add the chopped garlic, tarragon, sprinkle of salt, sprinkle of pepper and olive oil. Squeeze the lemon juice and zest in the bowl and mix everything together.

Add the salmon fillets to the bowl and coat them in the marinade. Cover the bowl and leave the salmon fillets to marinade for 10 minutes.

Take the salmon fillets out of the bowl and place on a tray, pouring the marinade over the top of the fillets.

Grill the salmon fillets for around 10 minutes or until cooked through.

Plate up and serve.

STRENGTHENING SUB-CONTINENTAL SARDINES

Sardines are a great source of protein as well as omega 3's.

CALORIES PER SERVING: 356

PROTEIN: 20G

CARBS: 52G

FAT: 7G

SERVES 4

50g plain flour

10 sardines, scaled and cleaned (8 if large)

Zest 2 lemons

Large bunch of chopped flat-leaf parsley,

3 garlic cloves, finely chopped

3 tbsp olive oil

400g of tinned chopped tomatoes

800g chickpeas or butterbeans, drained and rinsed

250g pack cherry tomatoes, halved

A pinch of salt and pepper

HOW TO MAKE:

Sprinkle the flour with salt and pepper and spread the flour out on the work surface.

Cover the sardines with the flour on each side.

Now in a separate bowl add the lemon zest to the chopped parsley (save a pinch for garnishing) and half of the chopped garlic, ready for later.

Put a very large pan on the grill and heat on high.

Now add the oil and once very hot, lay the floured sardines flat.

Fry for 3 minutes until golden underneath and turn over to fry for another 3 minutes. Put these onto a plate to rest.

Fry the remaining garlic (add another splash of oil if you need to) for 1 min until softened. Pour in the tin of chopped tomatoes, mix and let simmer for 4-5 minutes.

Tip in the chickpeas or butter beans and fresh tomatoes, then stir until heated through.

Here's when you add the sardines into the lemon and parsley mix and cook for a further 3-4 minutes.

Once they're cooked through, serve with a pinch of parsley to garnish.

SUPER TASTY COD PARCELS

A quick and easy muscle-building recipe to make: perfect for lunches or snacks.

CALORIES PER SERVING: 324

PROTEIN: 28G

CARBS: 11G

FAT: 19G

SERVES 2

2x 175g cod fillets

2 sheets of grease-proof or baking paper

2 tbsp chopped flat-leaf parsley

Juice of 1 lemon

175g organic cherry tomatoes

25g olives

1 tbsp olive oil

HOW TO MAKE:

Preheat oven to (180°C /350°f/Gas Mark 4).

Tear off a square of paper and place a cod fillet in the centre.

Scatter half of the other ingredients around it and fold shut.

Repeat with the other cod fillet.

Bake for 15 minutes in the oven.

Open the parcel and squeeze more lemon juice over to serve.

Plate and serve.

MIGHTY
TUNA MELTS

Not sure what to do with that tuna can at the back of the cupboard? This is a delicious protein pack recipe that's ready in minutes..

CALORIES PER SERVING: 450

PROTEIN: 37G

CARBS: 20G

FAT: 24G

SERVES 4

200g of tinned, drained tuna

Handful of chopped spring onions

4 tbsp low-fat mayonnaise

4 thick slices wholemeal bread

50g grated cheddar

2 tbsp of chilli flakes

1 squeezed lemon

A pinch of salt and pepper

HOW TO MAKE:

Toast the bread and pre-heat the grill.

Get a bowl and add the spring onions, mayonnaise, tuna and chilli flakes along with salt and pepper and the lemon juice. Mix everything together.

Spread the tuna mix over the top of the slices of bread and sprinkle the grated cheese over the top. Place under the grill until the cheese starts to bubble.

Plate up and serve.

TASTY TUNA,
BROCCOLI & CAULIFLOWER PASTA BAKE

Delicious pasta meal packed with protein for all your muscle-building and fat loss needs.

CALORIES PER SERVING: 641

PROTEIN: 37G

CARBS: 73G

FAT: 22G

SERVES 4

2 cans of tuna in olive oil (drained)

800g of canned chopped tomatoes

350g whole-wheat pasta

150g chopped broccoli

150g chopped cauliflower

200g pack light soft cheese

100g of grated cheddar

25g whole-wheat breadcrumbs

1 tbsp of Olive oil

HOW TO MAKE:

Grab a pan and heat the olive oil (medium/high heat).

Add the canned tomatoes and 200ml of water and let simmer.

Heat another large pan of water until it boils. Add the whole-wheat pasta and leave until the pan starts to boil again. Reduce the heat until the water simmers. Leave the whole-wheat pasta to cook for around 10 minutes. Add the broccoli and cauliflower during the last 3 minutes then drain.

Whilst the pasta and veg is cooking, pre heat the grill.

Add the cheese to the tomato sauce and stir until it melts, then add the drained pasta, vegetables and tuna.

Pour the mixture in a deep tray and cover with the cheddar, breadcrumbs, salt and pepper.

Place under the grill and cook for 6 minutes until golden.

Plate up and serve.

SUPERHUMAN
SEA BASS WITH SIZZLING SPICES

A delicious meaty meal that's packed full of protein.

CALORIES PER SERVING: 202

PROTEIN: 28G

CARBS: 2G

FAT: 9G

SERVES 6

6 x sea bass fillets skin on and scaled

3 tbsp olive oil

1 thumb-size piece of ginger, peeled and chopped into slices

3 thinly sliced garlic cloves

3 red chillies deseeded and thinly sliced

5 sliced spring onion stems

1 tbsp soy sauce

HOW TO MAKE:

Get a large pan and heat 2 tbsp of the oil on a medium heat.

Sprinkle salt and pepper over the Sea Bass and score the skin of the fish a few times with a sharp knife.

Add the sea bass fillet to the very hot pan with the skin side down (you must press the fish down onto the pan with your cooking spatula to prevent the fish from shrivelling and shrinking).

Cook the fish this way for around 5 minutes, or until you can see the skin underneath turning golden brown (you can lose the pressure on the spatula after the first few seconds)!

Now turn the fish over for around 30 seconds to give the flesh a nice golden colour.

Take the fish out of the pan, and place to one side.

Add the rest of the oil to the pan, throw in the chillies, garlic and ginger and cook for approximately 2 minutes or until golden.

Take this off the heat and add the spring onions with the soy sauce. Pour the sauce over your sea bass for a delicious oriental treat.

PROTEIN PACKED PAELLA

A delicious, traditional Spanish dish that's packed full over flavour and protein to ensure you continue to build muscle and burn fat.

CALORIES PER SERVING: 351

PROTEIN: 21G

CARBS: 50G

FAT: 9G

HOW TO MAKE:

Heat olive oil in a pan on a high heat. Add the chorizo, onion and garlic and then fry for 2-3 minutes until soft.

Add the turmeric, rice, prawns and frozen peas as well as 100ml of boiling water.

Stir until everything is warm and the water has been absorbed.

Plate up and serve.

SERVES 4

200g frozen cooked prawns

2 diced chorizo sausages

1 tbsp olive oil

1 chopped onion

1 chopped garlic clove

½ tsp turmeric

600g cooked brown rice

100g frozen peas

BRAWNY BAKED
HADDOCK WITH SPINACH AND PEA RISOTTO

Haddock is cheap and easy to cook and on top of this is packed full of nutrients and is a warm and wholesome filler!

CALORIES PER SERVING: 469

PROTEIN: 32G

CARBS: 66G

FAT: 10G

SERVES 4

400g skinless, boneless, smoked haddock from your local fishmonger or supermarket

1 tbsp olive oil

1 onion, chopped

300g risotto rice

450ml of vegetable stock

250g fresh spinach leaves

Handful of frozen peas

3 tbsp crème fraîche

50g grated parmesan cheese

A pinch of pepper

HOW TO MAKE:

Heat the oil in a large pan or wok on a medium heat.

Fry the chopped onion until just soft (not brown) before adding in the rice and stirring until soft.

Now add half of the stock and continue to stir slowly until the rice takes on a translucent texture.

Keep adding the rest of the stock slowly whilst stirring for up to 20-30 minutes.

Stir in the spinach and peas to the risotto.

Place the fish on top of the rice, replace the lid, then let steam for 10 minutes.

Flake the fish into large chunks and stir into the rice with the crème fraîche and half the parmesan.

Sprinkle with freshly ground pepper, then add the rest of the parmesan on top to taste!

RUSTIC
SCALLOPS WITH CORIANDER AND LIME

Scallops are a delicacy and if you feel like pushing the boat out, a great tasty change from the norm!

CALORIES PER SERVING: 225

PROTEIN: 20G

CARBS: 3G

FAT: 14G

HOW TO MAKE:

Heat pan on a medium to high and fry scallops for about 1 minute each side until golden. Add the chopped chilli and garlic cloves to the pan and squeeze the lime juice over the scallops.

Remove the scallops and sprinkle the chilli and coriander over them as well as some salt and pepper to serve.

SERVES 4

8 queen or king scallops (row on)

1 tbsp olive oil

2 large chopped garlic cloves

1 tsp chopped fresh red chilli

1/2 lime juice

2 tbsp of chopped coriander

A pinch of salt and pepper

TRAINING
TILAPIA IN THAI SAUCE

Tilapia is an exotic sounding fish but can often be found in your local fishmonger or superstore counter. Failing this, you can use this recipe with Sea bass or any other fish fillets of your choice!

CALORIES PER SERVING: 328

PROTEIN: 28G

CARBS: 25G

FAT: 14G

SERVES 4

4 tilapia fillets

2 tbsp flour

2 tbsp olive oil

4 spring onions, sliced

1 stick of chopped lemon grass

2 crushed garlic cloves

Small piece of chopped fresh ginger

2 tbsp soy sauce

Lime juice 1 lime, plus 1 lime chopped into wedges, to serve

1 chopped red chilli

Handful of coriander leaves

HOW TO MAKE:

Dip the tilapia fillets into the flour so that the whole fillet is coated.

Add olive oil to a pan on a medium to high heat and fry the fillets for 3 minutes on each side.

Using the same pan, fry the garlic, chilli, lemon grass and ginger on a low heat, adding the soy sauce and lime juice and simmering until the sauce thickens slightly.

Spoon the sauce over the fish and add the spring onions for a couple of minutes before dishing up and garnishing with your choice of herb and the lime wedges on the side.

TANGY
TROUT

Trout is the king of all river fish and its goodness cannot be underrated! Sea trout is just as majestic so don't rule it out!

CALORIES PER SERVING: 298

PROTEIN: 30G

CARBS: 10G

FAT: 16G

SERVES 4

4 trout fillets

50g whole wheat/brown breadcrumbs (you can buy these pre-packaged or just use your trusty blender to wiz up your crust ends!)

1 tbsp olive oil

1 small chopped bunch parsley

Zest and juice of 1 lemon

25g toasted and chopped pine nuts or walnuts

HOW TO MAKE:

Turn your grill up high.

In the meantime, spread a little oil over a baking tray and mix the breadcrumbs, parsley, lemon zest and juice and half of the nuts.

Lay the fillets skin side down onto your tray and rub into your mixture on both sides before drizzling with more olive oil.

Leave them under the grill for five minutes and then scatter over the rest of the nuts to serve.

STEAMY
WORKOUT FISH

This dish is fresh and delicious; it's so easy to cook and you can pack it full with extra greens and vitamins!

CALORIES PER SERVING: 145

PROTEIN: 29G

CARBS: 4G

FAT: 1G

SERVES 4

Tin foil, greaseproof paper or baking paper.

100g pak choi

4 x 150g fillets firm white fish (Cod, Plaice, Pollock, Seabass or Haddock)

2 garlic cloves, finely chopped

2 tbsp soy sauce

1 tsp mirin rice wine

4 chopped spring onions stems

HOW TO MAKE:

Heat oven to (200°C/400°F/Gas Mark 6).

You're going to be making a parcel for your delicious ingredients so you will need tin foil, greaseproof paper or baking paper.

Cut off four large rectangles and place each fillet on each piece of paper.

Add the garlic, soy sauce and rice wine.

You may want to use one or two of the lime wedges to squeeze the juices into your parcel.

Fold these up into a parcel leaving one edge open.

Cook for 20 minutes then add the spring onions and chilli for a fresh taste to end.

JOCK'S
JACKET POTATO WITH TUNA

Who said a jacket potato had to be boring? Try this sweet potato version and you'll be left satisfied and full with your fair share of protein!

CALORIES PER SERVING: 352

PROTEIN: 33G

CARBS: 27G

FAT: 13G

SERVES 1

1 large sweet potato

185g can tuna in olive oil, drained

½ finely chopped red onion,

1 small deseeded and chopped red chilli, (dried chilli will be just as good)

1 tbsp natural yoghurt

A bunch of chopped spring onions

HOW TO MAKE:

Preheat the oven to (200°C/400°F/Gas Mark 6).

You don't need to peel the sweet potato but you may want to scrape off the nobly bits with a sharp knife!

Pierce the potato with a fork multiple times and place in the microwave for 20 minutes (if you don't have a microwave you can use the oven but it will take around 30 minutes).

Whilst it's cooking, mix the tuna with the chopped onion and chill and season with salt and pepper.

Place the sweet potato in the pre-heated oven for a further 5-10 minutes or until a little crispy and serve with the tuna mix and yoghurt over the top.

Sprinkle the chopped spring onion over that!

SALADS

Salads are boring right? They're only designed for rabbits and skinny women on diets. Wrong. Salads done right are firstly delicious and don't have to just be a side; secondly they can be stuffed with fibre, protein, vitamins, nutrients. Don't make the stupid error of ignoring our trusted training companions and try a salad soon.

TUNA, SPINACH & QUINOA SALAD

Quick and easy tasty tuna salad for your muscle building and fat loss needs.

CALORIES PER SERVING: 302

PROTEIN: 18G

CARBS: 28G

FAT: 13G

SERVES 2

2 cans of tinned tuna in olive oil

Handful of baby spinach

1 chopped red onion

300g of chopped peppers

1 tbsp olive oil

1 chopped red chilli

225g of quinoa

350g of halved cherry tomatoes

1 cup of chopped black olives

HOW TO MAKE:

Add the quinoa to a large pan of boiling water and cook for 10 – 15 minutes until tender, then drain.

Heat oil in a pan on a medium heat and fry the onions, peppers and chilli until softened.

Get a bowl and add the drained quinoa, onion mix, tomatoes, tuna, baby spinach and olives and mix together.

Serve and enjoy

MEDITERRANEAN SUPER SALAD

Quinoa's goodness cannot be overstated, this salad is packed full of protein and is also delicious too.

CALORIES PER SERVING: 290

PROTEIN: 15G

CARBS: 35G

FAT: 10G

SERVES 1

200g quinoa

1 tsp olive oil

½ red onion, finely chopped

2 tbsp mint (fresh or dried) and roughly chopped

400g of Puy or red lentils rinsed and drained – you can buy the dried lentils but you need to leave them to soak over night.

¼ cucumber (skins off and diced)

100g crumbled feta cheese

Zest and juice of 1 orange

1 tbsp red or white wine vinegar

HOW TO MAKE:

Cook the quinoa in a large pan of boiling water for 10-15 minutes until soft, drain and set aside to cool.

Fry the onion in the oil over a medium heat.

Stir together with the quinoa, lentils, cucumber, feta, orange zest, chopped mint and juice and vinegar.

Best served chilled!

For the meat fans, cooked chicken or lamb would be a delicious addition to this dish!

HUNKED UP HALLOUMI

This cheese could almost be meat it's so chunky and filling!

CALORIES PER SERVING: 461

PROTEIN: 29G

CARBS: 3G

FAT: 37G

SERVES 4

2 tbsp white wine vinegar

1 tsp olive oil

½ red onion thinly sliced

Handful of rocket leaves

½ juiced lemon

Handful of green/black olives

500g of sliced halloumi cheese

1 tbsp mayonnaise

½ chopped cucumber

A pinch of pepper

HOW TO MAKE:

Preheat the grill.

Lightly drizzle a baking tray with 1 tsp olive oil before grilling for 5 minutes, turning until browned and crisp on the edges.

Add the chopped olives, rocket, cucumber and red onion into a bowl and mix with 1 tsp olive oil and lemon juice.

Season with pepper and stir in the mayonnaise (optional).

Serve alone or with crusty brown pitta breads for an Aegean twist!

ROASTED BEETROOT, GOATS CHEESE & EGG SALAD

Whether you love it or hate it, beetroot is a super food containing nutrients you rarely find in your five portions a day! Give it a go if you never have, or try this take on it if you're already a fan.

CALORIES PER SERVING: 363

PROTEIN: 11G

CARBS: 18G

FAT: 28G

SERVES 1

200g cooked chopped beetroot (not in vinegar)

2 tbsp olive oil

Juice from 1 orange

2 eggs

1 tsp white wine vinegar

2 tbsp crème fraîche

1 tsp Dijon mustard

A few stalks of dill, finely chopped (fresh or dried)

70g of baby gem lettuce

Handful of walnuts

100g crumbled goats cheese

A pinch of salt and pepper

HOW TO MAKE:

Preheat oven to (200°C/400°F/Gas Mark 6).

Place the beetroot onto the lightly oiled baking tray with the juice from the orange, sprinkle with salt and pepper.

Roast for 20-25 minutes, turning them once whilst they're baking. If they start to dry out, add a little more olive oil.

Meanwhile, put the eggs in boiling water. Turn down the heat and simmer for 8 minutes (4 minutes if you like your yolks runny) then run under cold water to cool. Peel and halve.

Mix the remaining oil, crème fraîche, mustard, a tsp of white wine vinegar and chopped dill together. This is the dressing for your lettuce.

Serve the salad with the beetroot and goats cheese crumbled over the top and walnuts sprinkled throughout.

SPICY MEXICAN BEAN STEW

This one is technically a salad but really it could pass on anyone's dinner table. You won't be left hungry after this one and you'll certainly feel the heat kick-starting your metabolism!

CALORIES PER SERVING: 395

PROTEIN: 20G

CARBS: 45G

FAT: 15G

SERVES 4

250g canned chick peas, drained

200g canned cannellini beans, drained

200g of tinned chopped tomatoes

2 tbsp olive oil

1 chopped red onion

190g of sliced chorizo

3 red chopped chillis

1 tbsp paprika

HOW TO MAKE:

Heat a large pan on a medium heat with 1 tbsp olive oil, and cook the onion and chorizo for 5 minutes until lightly golden.

Tip in the chickpeas with the cannellini beans and stir until heated through.

Add the tin of chopped tomatoes and paprika and cover to let simmer for 5-10 minutes.

Serve – recommended with crusty brown bread, couscous or brown rice for a winter warmer!

THE
SAILOR SALAD

Spinach was good enough for the well-known muscle-building sailor cartoon then and its more than good enough for you now; add a generous portion of the sailor's catch and you'll be growing bigger than he ever did.

CALORIES PER SERVING: 220

PROTEIN: 20G

CARBS: 12.5G

FAT: 10G

SERVES 4

2 cups of chopped spinach (fresh)*

170g of lean grilled chopped turkey breast (or turkey deli meat already cooked)

1tbsp real bacon bits (you can cut up bacon and grill this yourself or buy the pre-packaged stuff)

2 diced hard-boiled eggs

100g new/baby potatoes

1 deseeded and sliced red, yellow and green pepper

1 avocado peeled and sliced (do this near to the end or it will start to turn brown)

1 tbsp balsamic vinegar

HOW TO MAKE:

Boil a medium sized pan of water on a high heat and add the halved new potatoes, cooking for 15-20 minutes or according to packaging guidelines.

Combine the meats (once grilled and chopped if you're doing this yourself) with the spinach and peppers in a serving bowl.

Drain the potatoes and let cool whilst placing a small pan to boil for the eggs. Cook for 8 minutes for medium-boiled or 10 minutes for hard-boiled eggs.

Run the eggs under a cold tap and peel. Dice and add to your salad (here's where you can peel the avocado and add this).

Stir through with balsamic vinegar and salt and pepper to taste.

SIZZLING SALMON SALAD

Some like it hot. You can serve this one up with warm or cold salmon – either way it's wholesome and mouth-watering.

CALORIES PER SERVING: 521

PROTEIN: 46G

CARBS: 24G

FAT: 27G

SERVES 1

150g fillet salmon

6 cherry tomatoes

100g of couscous

3 stems of asparagus (chop off the very end of the base but leave the rest intact)

50g of diced low-fat mozzarella cheese

1 bell pepper sliced

1 tbsp balsamic vinegar

1 tbsp olive oil

A pinch of salt and pepper

HOW TO MAKE:

Preheat the grill.

Layer the couscous with boiling water from the kettle (about 1cm over the top of the couscous, cover and leave to steam)

Grill salmon for 10-15 minutes or until cooked through. Place to one side.

Uncover the couscous and stir through with a fork to break up the grains.

Now just add your pepper, mozzarella and halved cherry tomatoes to the couscous.

You will need to grill your asparagus for 3-4 minutes, turning every so often until lightly browned around the surface.

Once the asparagus is ready, place it along with the salmon on the bed of couscous and drizzle with olive oil and balsamic vinegar.

Salt and pepper to taste.

HERBY
TUNA STEAK

Protein, protein, protein!

SERVES 2

2x 200g dolphin-friendly yellow fin tuna steaks

1 tbsp olive oil

2 lemon wedges

2 handfuls of flat-leaf parsley and 2 handfuls of coriander very roughly chopped

2 cloves of finely chopped garlic

½ onion finely chopped

Handful chopped green olives

6 tbsp olive oil

50g pine nuts or walnuts

Juice of half a lemon

HOW TO MAKE:

Your first job is the herby salad – mix the herbs with half of the chopped garlic, lemon juice and olive oil.

Crush the nuts in a tea towel or blend them up in your blender. Stir them in to the herbs.

Brush the tuna steaks with olive oil and sprinkle with salt and pepper.

You need to heat dry pan to an extremely high heat (look out for the smoke)

Seal the tuna in the pan for one minute on each side (if you have a griddle pan or grill then you should place these against the lines to get that nice straight off the BBQ look and taste)

If you like your tuna less-pink cook for 2 minutes on each side for medium, 3 for medium well and 4 for well done (approximate times).

Once cooked serve straight away with your herby salad (pour this over as a dressing or on the side as an accompaniment)

MUSCLE BUILDING
STEAK & CHEESE SALAD

A very quick and easy, healthy muscle building salad.

CALORIES PER SERVING: 308

PROTEIN: 34G

CARBS: 15G

FAT: 14G

SERVES 2

250 frying beef steak

1 chopped red onion

1 teaspoon of crushed garlic

Handful of baby spinach

Handful of watercress

Handful of lettuce

4 chopped baby tomatoes

2 tbsp of balsamic vinegar

1 tbsp olive oil

50g of blue cheese

A pinch of salt and pepper

HOW TO MAKE:

Sprinkle salt and pepper over the steak.

Add a tbsp of olive oil to a griddle pan on a high heat.

Place the steak in the pan and cook 8 minutes in total, turning the steak half way through. Take the steak off the pan and allow to cool.

Cut the steak into 2cm strips, then place back into the pan and cook for a further minute on a medium heat.

Get a bowl and add the chopped tomatoes, watercress, baby spinach, lettuce, garlic and onions. Place the steak strips in the bowl along with the vinegar and a tbsp of olive oil. Mix everything together and grate the blue cheese over the top.

ANABOLIC
AVOCADO AND CHICKEN SALAD

A fresh and delicious salad, pleasing the meat eater and keeping you anabolic!

CALORIES PER SERVING: 389

PROTEIN: 36G

CARBS: 12G

FAT: 14G

SERVES 1

1 chicken breast

Handful of watercress

Handful of baby spinach

Handful of rocket

½ a sliced avocado

1 chopped Beef tomato

¼ sliced cucumber

2 tbsp of olive oil

HOW TO MAKE:

Heat some olive oil on a medium heat in a griddle pan.

Grill the chicken breast for about 10 minutes each side or until cooked through.

Cut the chicken breasts into chunks and serve with the watercress, spinach, rocket, tomato and sliced avocado.

Finish off the salad by drizzling over olive oil

STRENGTH
CHICKEN AND SESAME SALAD

Contains three sources of protein for all your muscle-building needs.

CALORIES PER SERVING: 430

PROTEIN: 20G

CARBS: 16G

FAT: 15G

SERVES 2

2 chicken breasts

3 tbsp of sesame oil

2 tsp of grated ginger

1 crushed garlic clove

1 chopped red chilli

1 diced red onion

Handful of basil leaves

Handful of coriander leaves

100g of baby spinach leaves

1 tsp of sesame seeds

4 chopped almonds

1 peeled and sliced mandarin

HOW TO MAKE:

Pre-heat the grill.

Add 2 tbsp sesame oil, chopped red chilli, crushed garlic and ginger into a bowl. Mix all the ingredients together.

Make a few deep cuts into the chicken breast and leave them to marinate in the mixture for roughly 3 hours.

Add the spinach leaves, coriander leaves, basil leaves, red onion, chopped almonds and sesame seeds to a bowl and mix together.

Remove the chicken and rub over the last of the marinade and grill for 10 minutes each side or until fully cooked.

Cut the chicken into strips and add to the salad bowl.

Add the mandarin to the bowl and drizzle 1 tbsp of sesame oil over the salad and serve.

SIDES

Not enough to fill you up? Craving your side order of fries? Eyes bigger than your belly? No sweat. Here's a sweet collection of side orders you can prepare in your own home – add calories, protein and a little extra something, whilst knowing you've made it in the healthy way.

SWEET POTATO WEDGES

Quick and easy. You won't be the only one devouring these tasty wedges.

CALORIES PER SERVING: 207

PROTEIN: 3G

CARBS: 38G

FAT: 6G

SERVES 4

4 sweet potatoes, scrubbed and cut into large wedges

2 tbsp olive oil

3-4 cloves of garlic

Handful of rosemary sprigs

HOW TO MAKE:

Pre-heat oven to (350°F/180 °C/Gas Mark 4).

Once you've scrubbed the skin of the sweet potatoes (don't remove it) with a kitchen scourer or something rough to suffice, you should toss the wedges in olive oil.

Spread these out on a baking tray, sprinkling the rosemary sprigs over the wedges and adding the whole garlic cloves in their skin over and around the wedges. Pop the whole lot into a pre-heated oven for 30-40 minutes or until crispy.

HOT & SPICY BUTTERNUT SQUASH

Often ignored in our fruit and veg selection, squash is a winner! One squash will feed a family, and if you're dining solo, freeze and save for another day!

CALORIES PER SERVING: 227

PROTEIN: 1G

CARBS: 30G

FAT: 14G

SERVES 4

1 butternut squash

4 tbsp olive oil

4 tbsp pouring honey

1 seeded and finely chopped red scotch bonnet chilli,

HOW TO MAKE:

Preheat the oven to (200°C/400°F/gas 6).

Chop the top and the bottom from the butternut squash. Next you need to cut it in half lengthways. You should now be able to use a vegetable peeler to remove the skin but if that doesn't work, take a sharp knife and cut downwards.

Now, using a spoon hollow out the seeds from the base.

You're free to slice now into thick (1-2 cm) slices horizontally.

On a lightly oiled baking tray, spread the slices into one layer across.

Drizzle the honey generously over the slices and sprinkle the chopped chili liberally (or according to heat tolerance!)

Bake for 35-40 minutes or until crispy.

Any left overs can be placed into a sealable sandwich bag and frozen – simply reheat in the oven when ready.

FRUITY NUTTY QUINOA

Don't know what to do with your quinoa? This dish is absolutely delicious and will go great with most main meals.

CALORIES PER SERVING: 328

PROTEIN: 10G

CARBS: 36G

FAT: 15G

HOW TO MAKE:

Add the quinoa to a large pan of boiling water and then let simmer for 10 – 15 minutes until tender, then drain.

Get a bowl and add the quinoa, apricots, herbs, lemon juice, zest and olive oil along with some salt and pepper and mix together.

Scatter the cashews over the top and serve.

SERVES 2

200g quinoa

6 dried apricots

Juice of 1 lemon

2 tbsp olive oil

A pinch of salt and pepper

Handful of chopped parsley and mint

50g cashew nuts

RICE & PEAS

Transport yourself to the Caribbean with this easy to prepare side dish.

CALORIES PER SERVING: 430

PROTEIN: 20G

CARBS: 16G

FAT: 15G

SERVES 2

300g brown rice

75ml olive oil

200g dried kidney beans

1 tsp chilli powder

HOW TO MAKE:

Soak the kidney beans in water overnight (you can buy tinned and use immediately if you're in a rush but you won't get that authentic color or taste!)

Boil the liquid with the kidney beans in using a large saucepan on a high heat (add water if you need to).

Add the rice and cook for 30 minutes and then drain. Keep the rice in the pan, add the kidney beans and cover and steam for 4 minutes.

Sprinkle chilli powder over your rice and serve

MUSCLE RICE SALAD

Add variety to your standard brown rice with this delicious and nutritious side..

CALORIES PER SERVING: 454

PROTEIN: 11G

CARBS: 64G

FAT: 19G

HOW TO MAKE:

Add 300ml of cold water to a pot and heat on high until the water is boiling.

Once boiling, add the rice and leave for 20 minutes. Then drain.

Mix the rice with chopped red pepper, chopped cucumber, grated carrot, cherry tomatoes and drizzle with olive oil.

SERVES 2

100g of brown rice

1 deseeded and finely chopped red pepper,

½ cucumber, deseeded and finely chopped

1 large grated carrot

1 cup of chopped cherry tomatoes

2 tbsp olive oil

LEMON & MOROCCAN MINT COUSCOUS

A fresh and zingy side dish that works well with fish, chicken, vegetables, even lamb and beef.

CALORIES PER SERVING: 367

PROTEIN: 6G

CARBS: 43G

FAT: 20G

SERVES 2

250g couscous

2 tbsp grated zest of a lemon and the lemon juice

20g pack fresh mint

4 tbsp toasted pine nuts

HOW TO MAKE:

In a serving bowl, pour boiling water over the dried couscous (it needs to cover the couscous with about a cm on the top) and cover the bowl with a plate to steam. You could add a chicken/vegetable stock cube to the boiling water for seasoning if you wish.

Once the couscous has steamed for a few minutes uncover it and use a fork to 'fluff up' the grains.

Add the lemon zest and juice, finely chopped mint and pine nuts.

Season to taste and add a little olive oil to serve.

MUSHROOM RISOTTO

Another dish that works well on the side – try it with chicken breast. Works great as a post workout side!

CALORIES PER SERVING: 445

PROTEIN: 15G

CARBS: 63G

FAT: 17G

SERVES 2

50g dried porcini mushrooms

1 vegetable stock cube

2 tbsp olive oil

1 finely chopped onion,

2 g finely chopped Garlic cloves,

250g sliced and washed pack chestnut mushrooms,

300g risotto rice, such as arborio

1 x 175ml white wine

Handful tarragon leaves chopped

50g freshly grated parmesan or grana padano,

HOW TO MAKE:

Pour 1 litre of boiling water over the dried porcini mushrooms and leave to soak for 20 minutes, then drain into a separate bowl (keep the liquid at this point as you need to add to the risotto later).

Chop the mushrooms into slices.

Heat up the oil on a medium heat in a large frying pan and add the onions and garlic, frying for around 5 minutes until they get soft.

At this point you should add the dried and fresh chestnut mushrooms and stir for another 5 minutes until softened.

Add the rice, stirring for a minute or so before adding all of the wine.

Let it get to simmering point (bubbling), and add a quarter of the mushroom stock.

Simmer the rice, stirring often, until the rice has absorbed all the liquid.

Keep adding the stock, a quarter at a time, each time waiting for the rice to absorb the liquid.

A lot of stirring is required until the rice is soft! If the liquid runs out and the rice is still a little hard you can continue to add small amounts of water.

When soft, take the pan off the heat and add half the cheese and tarragon leaves. Cover the pan and let it steam for a few minutes.

Serve with the rest of the cheese and herbs!

SWEDE & CARROT MASH UP

Try this home comfort – it's exciting mash!

CALORIES PER SERVING: 132

PROTEIN: 2G

CARBS: 22G

FAT: 5G

HOW TO MAKE:

Put the carrots, swede and garlic in a large pan of salted water, bring to the boil, and cook for 12 minutes. Add the tarragon and olive oil and season with salt and pepper.

Drain and then mash. Stir in a dollop of crème fraîche before serving if you like!

SERVES 4

500g chopped carrots

500g chopped swede

3 chopped garlic cloves

Handful of finely chopped tarragon,

1 tbsp olive oil

A pinch of salt and pepper

MUSTARDY CAULIFLOWER CHEESE

Winter Warmer – eat alone or on the side.

CALORIES PER SERVING: 240

PROTEIN: 15G

CARBS: 14G

FAT: 12G

SERVES 2

1 cauliflower

2 tbsp wholegrain mustard

100g mature cheddar cheese

100ml low-fat crème fraiche

HOW TO MAKE:

Chop the cauliflower by cutting off the thickest part of the stem and pulling apart the florets.

In a mixing bowl, place the cauliflower, ¾ of the cheese, crème fraîche and mustard and toss.

Place in an oven dish and pop into a preheated oven (200°C/400°F/gas 6) for 30 minutes.

Add the remaining cheese on to the top of the dish and grill for 5-7 minutes until brown and bubbling on top.

HOMEMADE PROTEIN SHAKES

If you want to spend hundreds of pounds on pre-made shakes full of chemicals and fillers that cements onto your kitchen sink then be my guest! If not, try these homemade healthy alternatives that will pack on just as much punch as the shop-bought varieties.

GREEN & MEAN

Begin your day with this easy to prepare veggie-rich breakfast that packs a monstrous protein-powered punch. Go Green!

CALORIES PER SERVING: 497

PROTEIN: 28

CARBS: 62

FAT: 17

HOW TO MAKE:

Place all the ingredients together in the blender and process until the desired consistency is achieved.

Pour contents of the blender into a tall glass. Serve immediately and enjoy!

SERVES 1

3 stalks of Celery

3 bunches of Kale

½ cup of sliced pineapple

½ apple, chopped

A handful of spinach

1 tbsp of coconut oil

1 scoop of vanilla protein powder

CHOCOLATE PEANUT DELIGHT

Get your chocolate fix with this tasty shake.

CALORIES PER SERVING: 656

PROTEIN: 63G

CARBS: 55G

FAT: 21G

HOW TO MAKE:

Add all the ingredients to a blender and blend until smooth.

Enjoy!

SERVES 1

1 scoop of chocolate whey protein powder

1 cup of low-fat Greek yogurt

1 whole banana

2 tbsp of peanut butter

1 cup of ice

JASON'S HOMEMADE MASS GAINER

It can be hard to get in the necessary calories to grow. Most weight gainers contain empty calories and can be expensive. This beast of a shake contains around 1000 healthy calories and a whopping 75g of Protein to keep you growing.

CALORIES PER SERVING: 970

PROTEIN: 75G

CARBS: 90G

FAT: 30G

HOW TO MAKE:

Add all the ingredients to a blender and blend until smooth.

Enjoy!

SERVES 1

2 scoop of chocolate whey protein powder

500ml of whole milk

55g of dry rolled oats

1 whole banana

2 tbsp of organic almond butter

1 cup of crushed ice

BERRY PROTEIN SHAKE

Totally refreshing on a hot summer's day and it works well any time of the year.

CALORIES PER SERVING: 342

PROTEIN: 38G

CARBS: 42G

FAT: 3G

HOW TO MAKE:

Add all the ingredients to a blender and blend until smooth.

Enjoy!

SERVES 1

2 scoop of whey protein powder

1 cup of blueberries

1 cup of blackberries

1 cup of raspberries

1 cup of water

1 cup of ice

FRESH
STRAWBERRY SHAKE

Keep it simple with this strawberry shake all year round

CALORIES PER SERVING: 303

PROTEIN: 35G

CARBS: 15G

FAT: 11G

HOW TO MAKE:

Add all the ingredients to a blender and blend until smooth.

Enjoy!

SERVES 1

2 scoops of vanilla protein powder

1 cup of strawberries

2 cups of water

1 tbsp of flaxseed oil

CHOCO
COFFEE ENERGY SHAKE

Swap your average morning caffeine hit with this refreshing alternative.

CALORIES PER SERVING: 299

PROTEIN: 42G

CARBS: 14G

FAT: 6G

HOW TO MAKE:

Add all the ingredients to a blender and blend until smooth.

Enjoy!

SERVES 1

2 scoops of chocolate protein powder

100ml of low-fat milk

1 cup of water

1 tbsp of instant coffee

LEAN AND MEAN PINEAPPLE SHAKE

Fresh, tropical and zingy – this shake really packs a punch and is crammed full with energy to keep you going until at least lunch -time.

CALORIES PER SERVING: 355

PROTEIN: 23G

CARBS: 65G

FAT: 3G

HOW TO MAKE:

Add all the ingredients to a blender and blend until smooth.

Enjoy!

SERVES 1

1 cup chopped pineapple

4 strawberries

1 banana

1 tbsp low-fat Greek yogurt

1 scoop of vanilla protein powder

1 cup of water

CHOPPED ALMOND SMOOTHIE

Quick and easy shake that will ease your chocolate craving and provide you with 24 grams of protein.

CALORIES PER SERVING: 241

PROTEIN: 24G

CARBS: 6G

FAT: 13G

HOW TO MAKE:

Add all the ingredients to a blender and blend until smooth.

Enjoy!

SERVES 1

1 1/2 cups water

17 chopped almonds

1/2 tsp coconut extract

1 scoop chocolate protein powder

VANILLA STRAWBERRY SURPRISE

If this doesn't transport you back to a day out by the seaside nothing will – it tastes amazing and is deceptively good at filling you up and helping you to bulk up and shred fat.

CALORIES PER SERVING: 329

PROTEIN: 36G

CARBS: 42G

FAT: 2G

HOW TO MAKE:

Add all the ingredients to a blender and blend until smooth.

Enjoy!

SERVES 1

2 scoops of vanilla protein powder

1 cup of ice

1 banana

4 fresh or frozen strawberries

BREAKFAST
BANANA SHAKE

Not much time? This breakfast shake packs a punch and will ensure a positive start to your day

CALORIES PER SERVING: 566

PROTEIN: 59G

CARBS: 69G

FAT: 6G

HOW TO MAKE:

Add all the ingredients to a blender and blend until smooth.

Enjoy!

SERVES 1

200ml low-fat milk

1 banana

100g of rolled oats

2 scoops of vanilla whey protein powder

PEACHY PUNCH

This peachy punch will satisfy your sweet tooth as well as providing 50 grams of protein.

CALORIES PER SERVING: 543

PROTEIN: 50G

CARBS: 57G

FAT: 11G

HOW TO MAKE:

Add all the ingredients to a blender and blend until smooth.

Enjoy!

SERVES 1

2 scoop of vanilla protein powder

200ml of low-fat milk

45g of rolled oats

1 chopped peach

1 cup of water

50g of low fat Greek yogurt

BLACKBERRY BRAWN

Quick and easy shake that is as tasty as it is nutritious.

CALORIES PER SERVING: 457

PROTEIN: 47G

CARBS: 30G

FAT: 16G

HOW TO MAKE:

Add all the ingredients to a blender and blend until smooth.

Enjoy!

SERVES 1

1 cup of blackberries

200ml of low–fat milk

2 tbsp of Flax Seed oil

50g of low-fat Greek yogurt

2 scoops of vanilla protein powder

1 Cup Ice

NO
WHEY!

No protein powder? This healthy, tasty shake contains a nice dose of protein to keep you growing!

CALORIES PER SERVING: 388

PROTEIN: 26G

CARBS: 32G

FAT: 22G

HOW TO MAKE:

Add all the ingredients to a blender and blend until smooth.

Enjoy!

SERVES 1

1 cup of blackberries

1 cup of strawberries

200ml of low-fat milk

130g of Greek yogurt

1 tbsp of almond butter

1 cup Ice

CARIBBEAN CRUSH

Absolutely delicious!

CALORIES PER SERVING: 263

PROTEIN: 25G

CARBS: 38G

FAT: 3G

HOW TO MAKE:

Add all the ingredients to a blender and blend until smooth.

Enjoy!

SERVES 1

1 scoop of protein powder (your choice)

1/2 chopped mango

1/2 cup of pineapple chunks

1 peeled and cubed kiwi

1 strawberry

1 cup of ice cubes

CHOCOLATE & RASPBERRY BANG

A tasty, quick protein shake to keep you growing and shredding!

CALORIES PER SERVING: 269

PROTEIN: 31G

CARBS: 16G

FAT: 9G

HOW TO MAKE:

Add all the ingredients to a blender and blend until smooth.

Enjoy!

SERVES 1

2 scoops of chocolate protein powder

1/2 cup of raspberries

200ml of whole milk

1/2 cup of ice cubes

CINNAMON SURPRISE

Quick and easy protein shake to satisfy your taste buds!

CALORIES PER SERVING: 244

PROTEIN: 47G

CARBS: 7G

FAT: 4G

HOW TO MAKE:

Add all the ingredients to a blender and blend until smooth.

Enjoy!

SERVES 1

2 scoops of chocolate protein powder

1 tbsp of cinnamon

1 cup of water

1 cup of ice

PUMPKIN POWER

A great tasting shake that's packed full of protein.

CALORIES PER SERVING: 224

PROTEIN: 38G

CARBS: 14G

FAT: 3G

HOW TO MAKE:

Add all the ingredients to a blender and blend until smooth.

Enjoy!

SERVES 1

2 scoops of vanilla protein powder

1 cup of chopped pumpkin

1 tsp cinnamon

1 cup of water

LIME POWER SHAKE

Bursting with Vitamin C goodness, this power shake is packed with muscle building protein as well!

CALORIES PER SERVING: 350

PROTEIN: 32G

CARBS: 52G

FAT: 6G

HOW TO MAKE:

Combine almond milk, protein powder, key lime juice, maple syrup, banana, and ice in the blender and process until smooth. Top the shake with graham cracker crumbs and a dollop of yogurt.

Serve in a tall glass!

SERVES 1

2 scoops of vanilla protein powder

1 piece of banana

1 cup of almond milk, unsweetened

1 tbsp of key lime juice

1 key lime zest

1 tbsp of non-fat Greek yogurt

1 tbsp of crushed graham crackers

1 cup of ice cubes

½ tsp of maple syrup

DESSERTS

Just because you are trying to build muscles doesn't mean you cannot indulge in sweet goodies once in a while. There are vegetarian desserts that are not only healthy, but rich in protein as well. Thus, your fitness goals will not be compromised. Here are some dessert recipes that you can try.

CHOCOLATE & PEANUT PUDDING PIE

A simple and easy recipe to make, this mouth-watering dessert is both cool and creamy. Even more, it is packed with a lot of muscle-boosting protein.

CALORIES PER SERVING: 322

PROTEIN: 20G

CARBS: 20G

FAT: 18G

HOW TO MAKE:

Mix the protein powder with pudding powder.

Stir the whipped cream and milk in until the mixture thickens.

Pour the mixture into the piecrust; allow it to cool in the refrigerator for half an hour.

Garnish with the peanut butter and walnuts. Serve and enjoy!

SERVES 1

1 pack of zero-fat, sugar-free chocolate pudding

250ml of not-fat milk

2 scoops of chocolate-flavored protein powder

3 tbsp of crunchy peanut butter

Handful of roasted walnuts

85g of whipped cream

1 piece of chocolate pie crust

JASON'S
PEANUT PROTEIN BARS

Save your money with these delicious, homemade protein bars!

CALORIES PER BAR: 386

PROTEIN: 18G

CARBS: 24G

FAT: 6G

MAKES 12 BARS

4 scoops of vanilla protein powder

400g of rolled oats

340g of almond butter

250ml of coconut cream

HOW TO MAKE:

Get a bowl and add the coconut cream and whisk until smooth, then add the protein powder and peanut butter and mix thoroughly.

Pour the oats into the bowl and again mix through.

Scoop out the mixture into a baking tray and flatten until the surface is smooth.

Place the tray in the fridge and leave for around 8 hours.

Cut into 12 bars.

POWER PARFAIT

A delicious dessert that tastes a great as it looks. Contains a whopping 38g of protein.

CALORIES PER SERVING: 254

PROTEIN: 38G

CARBS: 21G

FAT: 2G

HOW TO MAKE:

Mix the yogurt with the protein powder.

Get a tall parfait glass and layer with berries and yogurt.

SERVES 1

1 scoop of vanilla protein powder

2 cups of mixed berries

200ml of Greek yogurt

STRAWBERRY AND BANANA PROTEIN PUDDING

This is definitely a better alternative to yogurt-coated raisins. Though this simple recipe only has a few ingredients, it is not lacking in flavour and nutrients!

CALORIES PER SERVING: 195

PROTEIN: 23G

CARBS: 13G

FAT: 7G

SERVES 1

1 scoop of strawberry protein powder

60ml of egg whites

1 tbsp, non-fat, sugar-free chocolate pudding

3 pieces of strawberries, sliced

1 piece of small banana, sliced

Handful of blueberries

2 tbsp of water

HOW TO MAKE:

Combine the pudding and protein powder.

Add water and egg whites; mix well to achieve thick consistency.

Add powder if texture is still runny.

Spoon the batter out and transfer to a small plate.

Put in the freezer for half an hour.

Garnish with the strawberries, banana and blueberries

POWER PROTEIN WAFFLES

Who said waffles were unhealthy? Never mind, these are a great alternative

CALORIES PER SERVING: 314

PROTEIN: 37G

CARBS: 28G

FAT: 5G

HOW TO MAKE:

Add all the ingredients into a blender and blend.

Add the mixture to a waffle iron and bake.

SERVES 1

4 eggs whites

1 scoop of vanilla protein powder

40g of rolled oats

1 tsp of baking powder

½ tsp of stevia

BRAWNY BANANA PROTEIN COOKIES

This recipe is a must try recipe for banana lovers.

CALORIES PER SERVING: 359

PROTEIN: 25G

CARBS: 40G

FAT: 11G

SERVES 2

2 bananas

110g of oatmeal

2 scoop of vanilla protein powder

2 tsp of cinnamon

¼ tsp of baking powder

Handful of finely chopped walnuts or almonds

HOW TO MAKE:

Pre-heat the oven to 180C/350F/Gas Mark 4.

Oil-spray a non-stick pan.

Lightly oil-spray a cookie sheet. Distribute the oil evenly using a paper towel.

Get a large-sized bowl and mash the bananas until a creamy texture is achieved.

Add protein powder, oat, salt, walnuts, baking powder, and cinnamon. Mix well. Spoon mixture onto cookie sheet, forming cookie shaped pieces.

Bake for around 15 minutes.

Serve.

GREEK YOGURT WITH HONEY AND BERRIES

A quick and easy dessert that contains a whopping 43g of protein. .

CALORIES PER SERVING: 522

PROTEIN: 43G

CARBS: 86G

FAT: 7G

HOW TO MAKE:

Mix all your ingredients and you've got a fresh and healthy dessert with nothing on your conscience. You could sprinkle flaked almonds over the top for a bit of crunch.

SERVES 1

1 scoop of vanilla protein powder

100g Greek Yoghurt

4 tbsp of honey

45g of berries

POWER
PEANUT CHOCOLATE PANCAKES

Quick and easy great recipe. Contains lots of protein to keep you anabolic and is also low on carbs.

CALORIES PER SERVING: 286

PROTEIN: 33G

CARBS: 16G

FAT: 10G

HOW TO MAKE:

Get a bowl and combine all ingredients. Mix well until you get a thick batter.

Pour the butter on a greased skillet like you would a pancake, frying over a medium heat.

Serve when done cooking.

SERVES 2

1 scoop of chocolate protein powder

1 tbsp of smooth peanut butter

2 egg whites

2 tbsp of raw coconut flour

STRENGTH STRAWBERRY & CHEESE SURPRISE

Another heavenly combination – blueberry and cheese – this is a must-try vegetarian version, especially for muscle builders

CALORIES PER SERVING: 167

PROTEIN: 15G

CARBS: 20G

FAT: 3G

SERVES 4

110g of low-fat cottage cheese

80g of whole strawberry, fresh

60ml of egg whites

60ml of skim milk

100g of whole wheat flour

1 packet of stevia

1 ½ tsp of lemon juice

HOW TO MAKE:

Combine the skim milk, flour, and cottage cheese in a mixing bowl.

Beat the egg whites to get frothy consistency. Add to cheese mixture.

Stir in lemon juice. Toss in the strawberries. Stir again.

Transfer the batter into a non-stick frying pan. Turn when the tops start to bubble, and the bottom part starts to turn brown.

Serve.

PROTEIN
PUMPKIN COOKIES

Caving for cookies? This easy low-fat recipe is sure to give you a healthy fix.

CALORIES PER SERVING: 136

PROTEIN: 10G

CARBS: 15G

FAT: 4G

SERVES 4

2 scoops of vanilla protein powder

2 boxes of spice cake mix

150g of chocolate chips

700g of pumpkin (1 can)

HOW TO MAKE:

Pre-heat the oven to 180C/350F/Gas Mark 4.

Oil-spray a non-stick pan.

Lightly oil-spray a cookie sheet. Distribute the oil evenly using a paper towel.

Get a large-sized bowl and mash the bananas until a creamy texture is achieved.

Add protein powder, oat, salt, walnuts, baking powder, and cinnamon. Mix well. Spoon mixture onto cookie sheet, forming cookie shaped pieces.

Bake for around 15 minutes.

Serve.

COTTAGE CHEESECAKE

A hearty, protein packed cheesecake to enjoy!

CALORIES PER SERVING: 487

PROTEIN: 43G

CARBS: 53G

FAT: 7G

HOW TO MAKE:

Add all the ingredients to a blender and blend until smooth.

Place in a bowl and top with the strawberries.

Place in the fridge for 20 minutes.

SERVES 1

150g of fat free cottage cheese

1 scoop of vanilla protein powder

1 packet of stevia

1 tbsp sugar free instant pudding mix

5 tbsp of low fat milk

Handful of Strawberries

CONVERSION CHARTS

Volume

Imperial	Metric
1 tbsp	15ml
2 fl oz	55 ml
3 fl oz	75 ml
5 fl oz (¼ pint)	150 ml
10 fl oz (½ pint)	275 ml
1 pint	570 ml
1 ¼ pints	725 ml
1 ¾ pints	1 litre
2 pints	1.2 litres
2½ pints	1.5 litres
4 pints	2.25 litres

Weight

Imperial	Metric
½ oz	10 g
¾ oz	20 g
1 oz	25 g
1½ oz	40 g
2 oz	50 g
2½ oz	60 g
3 oz	75 g
4 oz	110 g
4½ oz	125 g
5 oz	150 g
6 oz	175 g
7 oz	200 g
8 oz	225 g
9 oz	250 g
10 oz	275 g
12 oz	350 g
1 lb	450 g
1 lb 8 oz	700 g
2 lb	900 g
3 lb	1.35 kg

Cups	Imperial	Metric
1 cup flour	5oz	150g
1 cup caster or granulated sugar	8oz	225g
1 cup soft brown sugar	6oz	175g
1 cup soft butter/margarine	8oz	225g
1 cup sultanas/raisins	7oz	200g
1 cup currants	5oz	150g
1 cup ground almonds	4oz	110g
1 cup oats	4oz	110g
1 cup golden syrup/honey	12oz	350g
1 cup uncooked rice	7oz	200g
1 cup grated cheese	4oz	110g
1 stick butter	4oz	110g
¼ cup liquid (water, milk, oil etc)	4 tablespoons	60ml
½ cup liquid (water, milk, oil etc)	¼ pint	125ml
1 cup liquid (water, milk, oil etc)	½ pint	250ml

Oven temperatures

Gas Mark	Fahrenheit	Celsius
1/4	225	110
1/2	250	130
1	275	140
2	300	150
3	325	170
4	350	180
5	375	190
6	400	200
7	425	220
8	450	230
9	475	240

BONUS CONTENT:

THE FAST AND FRESH
BODYBUILDING COOKBOOK MEAL PLANS
(100% FREE)

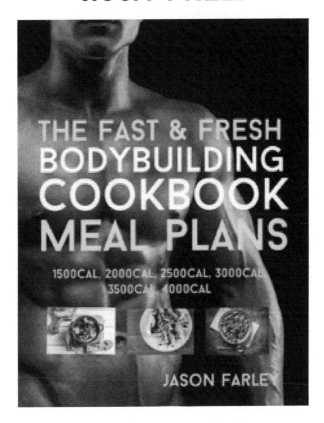

I believe that anyone can build a fantastic body and to ensure you get there, I created
The Fast and Fresh Bodybuilding Cookbook Meal Plans as a counterpart to this cookbook to save you the
hard work when it comes to what to eat, how much to eat and when to eat.

This special manual contains 6 different delicious daily meal plans ranging from 1500 calories all the way to a
whopping 4000 calories, so you're in control of how big or shredded you wanna get!

VISIT : HTTP://BIT.LY/FASTANDFRESHMEALPLANS
TO GET THIS NOW!

WOULD YOU MIND DOING ME A FAVOR?

Thanks again for purchasing my book. I'm confident that you'll love the recipes and hope that they will help you in your quest to burn fat and build more muscle!

Before you leave, I have a little favor to ask. If you enjoyed this book, would you mind taking a minute to write a brief blurb about this book on Amazon? I love to get feedback on my work and I would be really grateful!

Also if you have any questions regarding health / fitness or nutrition, feel free to get in touch. I'd love to help!

Feel free to send an email to **jason_farley@buffgains.com**
or check out my website: **www.buffgains.com** for more content!

All the best!

Jason

OTHER BOOKS BY ME...

I've been training for over a decade now. Getting in shape can be a hard task with so much misinformation, myths, scams and just plain B.S thrown around in the fitness industry. I see so many people fall for the same false promises every day.

With my books, I want to educate and support you in your quest to achieve all of your fitness goals. Whether you want to build muscle or burn fat and get shred-ded, there's something here for you. All of my books provide proven, sound train-ing and nutritional advice backed by science (no bro-science here!)

And you won't need a fancy gym membership, tons of money or expensive supplements to be successful with my books - just the desire and willpower to change your life!

I hope you like my books and I look forward to hearing about your amazing transformation!

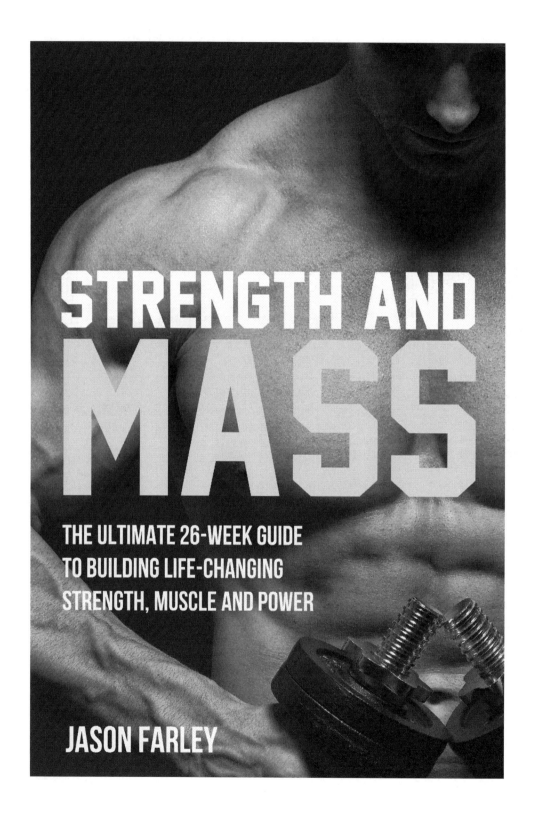

STRENGTH AND MASS

THE ULTIMATE 26-WEEK GUIDE TO BUILDING LIFE-CHANGING STRENGTH, MUSCLE AND POWER

JASON FARLEY

If you want to possess a lean, muscular and strong physique that demands respect and attention wherever you go...without wasting money on worthless supplements or steroids...then STRENGTH AND MASS is your answer.

I'm sure you've wondered what it takes to build a truly unbelievable body. The kind that women love and men envy...

I bet you've asked yourself questions like ...

"What exercises should I be doing?"
"How many days a week should I be training?"
"How many calories should I be eating?"

Well, in this book you're going to learn the answers to these and much, much more.

Strength and Mass is a step-by-step muscle-building program designed to improve size, strength and power without putting on unnecessary body fat. Within these pages, you'll finally learn exactly what it takes to build the body of your dreams.

Strength and Mass includes...

• A comprehensive, detailed and structured 26 week muscle building program – You will be told exactly how many reps, sets and exercises to do and when to do them.
• A fully detailed nutrition guide – You will be given full macronutrient breakdowns and a complete formula for calculating how many calories you need to grow!

And much much more!

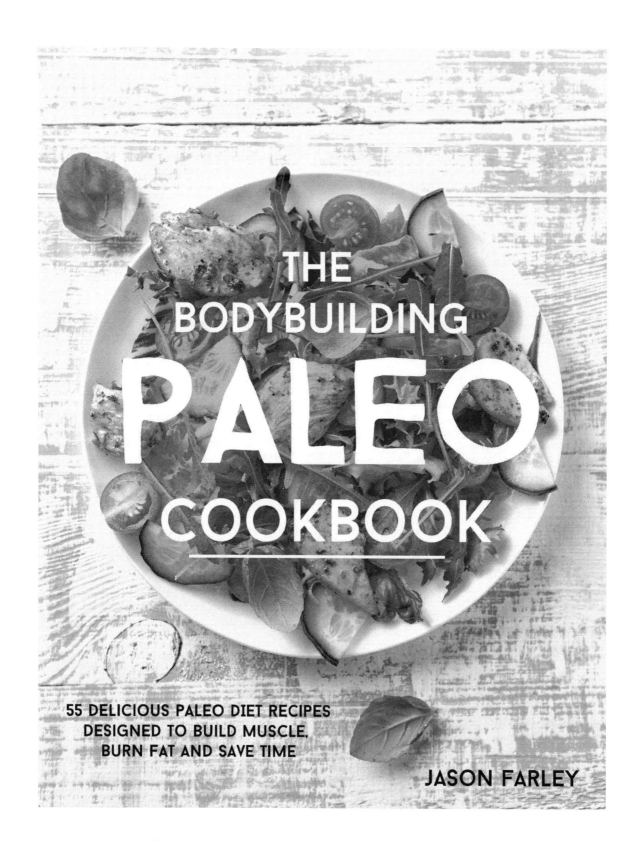

THE
BODYBUILDING
PALEO
COOKBOOK

55 DELICIOUS PALEO DIET RECIPES
DESIGNED TO BUILD MUSCLE,
BURN FAT AND SAVE TIME

JASON FARLEY

If you want to learn how to create healthy, delicious and nutritious paleo meals that are specially designed to build muscle, burn fat and save time, then THE BODYBUILDING PALEO COOKBOOK is your answer!

Every serious athlete knows that your nutrition is the most crucial part of building a lean, muscular and strong physique and can either make or break the results you see in the gym. However keeping to a paleo diet while training can be extremely difficult as so many foods are just off limits. This can make things really tough, especially when you need to get in a certain amount of calories and fuel your demanding workouts in the gym!

And lets face it…

Most Paleo recipes are just downright bland and boring!

With The Bodybuilding Paleo Cookbook, you'll never have to be frustrated with your paleo diet again. You'll learn how to cook tasty, quick and easy paleo meals that will build quality lean muscle mass, burn fat fast and save time. Every recipe included in this cookbook has been meticulous designed with the right macronutrient profile (protein, fats & carbs) to ensure that you reach your training goals!

And in case you were wondering, these recipes aren't just a slight upgrade to the standard paleo recipes like you'd find in most other cookbooks. These recipes are so delicious that you won't miss "regular" meals!

The Bodybuilding Paleo Cookbook includes…

• 7 mouth-watering breakfast meals like my Warrior Steak and Egg Supreme, Caveman Red Pepper Chicken Omelette, Action Avocado and Bacon Boost and Spiced Pumpkin Pancakes. They will kick-start your engine and ensure you start off the day as you mean to go on!

• 10 succulent and delicious chicken and poultry recipes like my Sweet Honey Chicken, Super Sticky Chicken Clubs and Grilled Chicken Kebabs. Say bye bye to boiled bland chicken. These meals will ensure that your body has no choice but to burn fat and build muscle!

And much, much more…

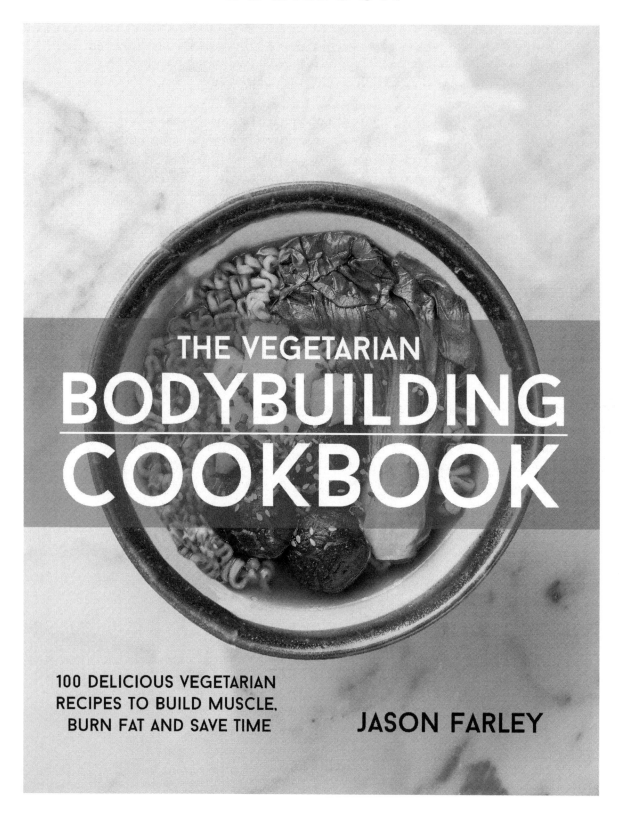

THE VEGETARIAN
BODYBUILDING
COOKBOOK

100 DELICIOUS VEGETARIAN
RECIPES TO BUILD MUSCLE,
BURN FAT AND SAVE TIME

JASON FARLEY

If you want to learn how to create healthy, delicious and nutritious vegetarian meals that are specially designed to build muscle, burn fat and save time, then THE VEGETARIAN BODYBUILDING COOKBOOK is your answer!

Every serious athlete knows that your nutrition is the most crucial part of building a lean, muscular and strong physique and can either make or break the results you see in the gym. However building muscle on a vegetarian diet can be more difficult as many foods are off limits. This can make things really tough, especially when you need to get in a certain amount of calories and fuel your demanding workouts in the gym!

And lets face it…

Most Vegetarian bodybuilding recipes are just downright bland and boring!

With The Vegetarian Bodybuilding Cookbook, you'll never have to be frustrated with your diet again. You'll learn how to cook healthy, tasty, quick and easy meals that will build quality lean muscle mass, burn fat fast and won't cost you an arm and a leg!

And these recipes aren't just a slight upgrade to familiar bodybuilding meals like you'd find in most health and fitness cookbooks. These recipes are so delicious your taste buds will believe you're in a 5 star restaurant!

The Vegetarian Bodybuilding Cookbook includes…

• 19 mouth-watering breakfast meals like my Muscle Fruit & Nut cereal , Lean & Mean Veggie Burger, Oat Muscle Mush and Brawny Veggie Sausage Club. They will kick-start your engine and ensure you start off the day as you mean to go on!

• 20 succulent and delicious entrees recipes like my Veggie Brawn Burger, Speedy Black Bean Surprise, Brawny Veg Lasagna, Tofu Lettuce Wraps and Feta & Brawny Barley Stuffed Portabellas. These meals will ensure that your body has no choice but to burn fat and build muscle!

• 19 gourmet snacks like my Muscle Feta Cheese & Olives, Quick Fix Roasted Beans, Protein Packed Latte and Sweet Potato Wedges.

• 13 tasty and nutritious sides like my Brawny Guacamole Hummus, Kale dip,

Made in the USA
Lexington, KY
13 May 2019